Holistic Health
Through Macrobiotics

Holistic Health Through Macrobiotics

A Complete Guide to Mind/Body Healing

Michio Kushi
with Edward Esko

Japan Publications, Inc.
Tokyo • New York

Note to the reader: Those with health problems are advised to seek the guidance of a qualified medical or psychological professional in addition to a qualified macrobiotic teacher before implementing any of the dietary or other approaches presented in this book. It is essential that any reader who has any reason to suspect serious illness seek appropriate medical, nutritional, or psychological advice promptly. Neither this nor any other related book should be used as a substitute for qualified care or treatment.

Published by Japan Publications, Inc., Tokyo and New York

Distributors:
UNITED STATES: Kodansha America, Inc., through Farrar, Straus & Giroux, 19 Union Square West, New York, N.Y. 10003. CANADA: Fitzhenry & Whiteside Ltd., 195 Allstate Parkway, Markham, Ontario L3R 4T8. BRITISH ISLES AND EUROPEAN CONTINENT: Premier Book Marketing Ltd., 1 Gower Street, London WC1E6HA. AUSTRALIA AND NEW ZEALAND: Bookwise International, 54 Crittenden Road, Findon, South Australia 5023. THE FAR EAST AND JAPAN: Japan Publications Trading Co., Ltd., 1–2–1, Sarugaku-cho, Chiyoda-ku, Tokyo 101.

First Edition: November 1993
LCCC: 93–078191
ISBN: 0–87040–895–X

Preface

Spiritual awakening is the most important issue in health and healing. Self-reflection, leading to an awareness of the endless order of the universe, is the basis for healing the body, mind, and spirit. Self-reflection leads us to abandon self-destructive habits and bring our way of eating and living into greater harmony with nature. A centrally-balanced, macrobiotic diet based on whole cereal grains, beans, fresh local vegetables, and other whole natural foods is the most basic reflection of a way of life in harmony with nature. A naturally balanced diet provides the biological foundation for genuine health, while the spiritual foundation is provided by a deep sense of gratitude toward nature, the universe, and life itself.

A peaceful mind is fundamental to achieving good health. It is important to minimize stress and relax mentally and physically. Holistic healing encourages everyone to have a peaceful mind and a positive attitude toward life. However, in today's society, when a person develops a chronic illness, he may receive a negative prognosis from his doctor. A negative prognosis has the opposite effect. It limits a person's freedom and causes stress and anxiety. It can have a negative effect on the outcome of an illness. In order to overcome a negative prognosis, it is important for a person to keep a positive image of the future while at the same time taking constructive steps to change his way of life. Making an optimistic plan for the future can be very helpful in this regard.

The quality of our environment also has a powerful effect on our health. A natural, non-toxic environment supports the process of healing, while an artificial, toxic environment limits it.

cess of healing, while an artificial, toxic environment limits it. Such things as concrete buildings, fluorescent lights, the artificial materials used in clothing and home furnishings, and the constant vibration of televisions, air conditioners, computers, electric stoves, and microwave ovens disrupts the natural flow of healing energy. It is important to live as close to nature as possible. A regular daily life, in which we live in harmony with the cycle of day and night by being active during the day and getting adequate rest at night, enhances the recovery of health. Eating regular meals and keeping a reasonable daily schedule also helps to restore harmony in body and mind.

Our health depends on the active flow of blood and energy throughout the body. A daily half-hour walk helps activate circulation, and is highly recommended. Other types of exercise are fine if they are enjoyable. However, it is not necessary to exercise to the point of exhaustion. If a person is unable to walk for an extended period, simply getting outside in the fresh air for ten minutes every day is helpful. Daily body scrubbing also activates blood and energy flow, as do practices such as Do-In and shiatsu massage, all of which are described in this book.

In some cases, these measures are sufficient to restore health. In others, simple, natural home remedies may be necessary for a short time until balance is restored. These include internal and external preparations such as special dishes, drinks, and plasters made from daily foods. The highest quality home remedies are easy to prepare at home, inexpensive, non-toxic, yet highly effective. All of the home remedies described in this book are prepared from common daily foods and fulfill these criteria.

Self-reflection and spiritual awakening cannot be provided by someone else. They are a product of our own self-realization and practice. Things such as how to balance daily food and how to make our environment and activity health-supporting can be learned from others, as can basic home remedies and simple energy treatments.

Ideally, however, once the basic principles of healthful living have been learned, a person should be able to manage daily health practices on his own without having to depend on someone else. Holistic healing thus encourages self-reliance and the self-management of health.

The origin of sickness is our view of life. Therefore, holistic healing begins with the central issues—spiritual awakening and self-realization, together with daily diet and activity—and employs peripheral symptomatic techniques only when necessary. The holistic approach is opposite to that of conventional medicine, which begins with symptomatic techniques while leaving these central issues completely untouched. It is for this reason that conventional medicine has been unable to stem the rise of degenerative disease.

Spiritual awakening is based on an awareness of our innate human freedom, including an understanding of how we create sickness and unhappiness through our thinking and behavior, and how we can change our condition toward genuine health. The purpose of holistic healing is to guide everyone toward self-realization and the free management of their health and their life. The central issues in health and healing—self-reflection and self-realization—are completely free, while the techniques employed by our current health care system are often very expensive. Ideally, health should be the product of daily life itself, including our way of thinking, diet, and activity. The way to health should be simple rather than complicated, affordable rather than expensive, and accessible to everyone as a part of day-to-day living. Moreover, the way to personal health should be the same as the way to social and planetary health. Creating a healthy and peaceful future for all people on earth is actually the goal of holistic macrobiotic healing.

In this book we discuss the central issues in health and healing, beginning with principles that can unify alternative and conventional, traditional and modern, and Eastern and Western approaches to health care. We discuss the unity of mind and body, and the effect that our way of thinking, diet, and activity have on our health and happiness. We explain the process of healing according to the traditional Oriental concept of Ki or energy, and discuss how healing is primarily an energetic phenomenon. We also discuss traditional Oriental macrobiotic diagnosis, the principles and practice of the macrobiotic diet, the use of daily food as medicine, and macrobiotic home remedies.

We would like to thank everyone who participated in the creation of this book. We especially wish to extend our gratitude to Iwao Yoshizaki, the former president of Japan Publications, Inc., for inspiring the creation of this book. Mr. Yoshizaki, who passed away last autumn, was a personal friend and a pioneer in macrobiotic publishing. Following his vision, Japan Publications, Inc., took the lead in publishing a wide variety of books on macrobiotics, Oriental medicine and philosophy, and holistic health. Mr. Yoshizaki was truly a citizen of one world, and we hope that this book will contribute to his dream of planetary health and peace.

We would also like to thank Yoshiro Fujiwara, the New York representative of Japan Publications, Inc., for his encouragement and support. We thank Alex Jack of One Peaceful World Press in Becket for supervising the production of the book, and Gale Jack for copyediting the manuscript. We also thank Wendy Esko and Lynda Shoup for their inspiration and support, and Bettina Zumdick for contributing illustrations for the book.

Michio Kushi
Edward Esko
Becket, Massachusetts
April, 1993

Contents

1
Holistic Perspectives

Today we are in need of principles that unify Eastern and Western, ancient and modern, spiritual and scientific, and holistic and analytical approaches to health and healing. As Norman Cousins states in *Anatomy of an Illness*:

> At the various holistic health conferences I attended, I became aware of a troubling contradiction. A movement based on the concept of wholeness was itself becoming unwhole. Two dozen or more schools or approaches of varying validity, not all of them compatible and some of them competitive, were crowding the center of the holistic stage. Some conferences on holistic health seemed more like a congeries of exhibits and separate theories than the occasion for articulating a cohesive philosophy.

In *Health and Healing: Understanding Conventional and Alternative Medicine*, Andrew Weil, M.D. alludes to a similar problem in modern allopathic medicine:

> Lacking a clear and unified theory, allopathy is a vast and cumbersome body of data concerning the identification of specific, physical agents of disease and the use of particular treatments directed against those agents. One consequence of this deficiency in theory is the difficulty of teaching the sys-

tem. Medical school curriculums are notoriously unwieldy and inefficient because teachers have to expose students to endless facts and details. If they could teach a basic conceptual framework on which to organize the details, medical teaching could be simplified greatly.

In this chapter, we introduce a set of comprehensive principles that, if properly understood and applied, could unify the varied approaches to health and healing, both past and present, found throughout the world. These principles derive from an understanding of natural law, and apply not only to healing, but to all areas of life. In the sections that follow, we explore these principles in depth.

Unity in Diversity

All things in the universe share certain fundamental characteristics. Let us take as examples common objects such as a pencil, desk, book, and plant. Each of these objects exists within time and space; they all have this in common. Moreover, since they exist on earth at the present time, they share an infinitesimally small segment of the time-space continuum. They all have a physical form defined by such things as shape, size, color, weight, and density, and are formed by the coming together of atoms and molecules. At the same time, they will eventually decompose through the separation of these components. The atoms that comprise each object are all in a constant state of motion, and each object will ultimately change form. In that sense, each thing is ephemeral, existing for only a brief period within the endless ocean of time.

Attributes such as these are common to all things, from galaxies to atoms, stars to cells, water vapor to diamonds, and elephants to bacteria. All things share a common origin—the universe—and pass through a life cycle defined by a beginning, middle, and end, followed by a new beginning in a different form. Everything is constantly moving and changing.

However, even though all things have certain characteristics in common, no two things are identical. Each is a unique manifestation of the universe. Perfect "sameness" does not exist. Things come into being and exist within time and space, yet no two occupy the same position in time and space. While all physical objects are made up of atoms and molecules, the number and combination of atoms and molecules is unique in each.

Returning to the four objects cited above, we see that although they all have color, texture, shape, density, and weight, these attributes are different in each. Although they are all produced by materials found on earth, the materials that comprise each are different, as are the methods involved in their creation. The pencil, table, and book are man-made, while the plant is created by nature. Each of the man-made objects is composed of wood, yet each is made of wood taken from a different tree, and processed in a different way. Each of these objects has some type of use, yet each is used differently. Each has value, yet the value of each is different.

Human beings are perfect examples of the principle of unity in diversity. If we compare any two people, we see that in comparison to other things, they look alike and move in pretty much the same way. In other words, they have a similar form and pattern of movement. They also share basic biological functions such as breathing, eating, discharging waste, sleeping, and reproduction. They also have a similar life pattern, beginning with birth, proceeding through growth, maturity, old age, and ending at death. Both have a mother, father, and ancestors stretching back through time. Moreover, they share a common environment, the earth, within a common time period, the latter part of the twentieth century. Both have been exposed to the values, concepts, and lifestyles that characterize modern civilization. They probably have read many of the same books, seen the same movies, watched the same television programs, and eaten the same types of foods. Both have basic physical needs, for example, for food, clothing, shelter, activity, and rest, and emotional needs such as the need for love, acceptance, friendship, and a sense of being part of a larger group. Both have a visible, physical nature, along with an invisible mental and spiritual nature. Like everyone else, both are seeking happiness and fulfillment in life.

However, even though people share certain basic characteristics, each person is completely unique. Each is born at a different time and in a different place, and each has a different size, weight, body build, facial features, hair color, and genetic make-up. Although human beings share basic life functions, each person has a different appetite and food preferences, each breathes in a different way, each pursues a different type and level of activity, and each needs a specific amount of rest. Although the pattern of life is potentially the same for all people, the way this pattern plays out differs from person to person. We all share a common environment, the earth, yet each of us occupies a different portion of that environment. Although each person has eyes, ears, skin, and other sensory organs, each perceives the environment in a slightly different way. Similarly, although people today are living within modern civilization, the influence that each person receives from society depends on such variables as family background, place of birth, education, travel, reading, and a multitude of others. And although the pursuit of happiness is common to everyone, each person has his or her own definition of happiness.

Polarity

One characteristic that all things have in common is that they are made up of numerous polarities. A chair, for example, is comprised of legs that project downward and a seat that extends upward in the opposite direction. Each section of the chair—and the chair as a whole—contains an upper and lower part, a left and right side, a top and bottom, and an inside and outside. The polarities in each of these pairs complement one another, and each pair of polarities is complementary to all the others. Together they comprise the unity that makes up the chair.

Numerous polarities exist in a book. Books are composed of

an outside and inside, a cover and contents. Their front and back covers complement one another: the front cover is usually bold and direct, while the back cover is understated and detailed. When we open a book, it divides into left and right-hand pages, and each page has a front and a back side. The book itself is defined by the polarity between its left- and right and upper and lower borders, its first and last pages, and its beginning and end. The pages of the book contain text and illustrations, printed type and blank space, headings and text, words and punctuation, letters and numbers, vowels and consonants, nouns and verbs, subjects and objects, and many other pairs of polarities.

The laws of economics, which govern the production and distribution of books and other consumer goods, are also driven by polarities. Economic activity is governed by the interplay between such things as supply and demand, income and expense, and producer and consumer. In order to compete successfully in the modern economy, producers must keep their costs as low as possible, while charging the highest possible price for their products. Consumers approach the marketplace from the opposite direction. They would like to see manufacturers spend as much as possible producing high-quality products while paying as little as possible for them.

Books, like everything else, do not exist in isolation. They exist in relation to other things in the environment and to the environment as a whole. These relationships are also defined by polarities. If we compare books, for example, we see that some are thick, others thin, some are colorful, others plain, some are large, others small, some are interesting, others dull, some are read by many people, others by few. Polarities also distinguish books from other objects, and make things appear distinct from the environment as a whole.

The biological world is also based on polarity. Complementary distinctions exist between plants and animals, more developed and less developed species, and creatures that live in water and those living on land. Some living things lay eggs, others carry their young inside their bodies, some eat plants, others are carnivorous, and some, like giant redwoods, live for centuries, while others, such as fruit flies, live for only several hours. Numerous polarities can be found within the structure and function of each living thing. If we take the human body as an example, we see that it has a left and right side, an upper and lower portion, a front and back, an inside and outside. The twin branches of the autonomic nervous system—the sympathetic and parasympathetic—work in an antagonistic, yet complementary manner to control the body's automatic functions. The endocrine system operates in a similar way. The pancreas secretes insulin, which lowers the blood sugar level, and also secretes anti-insulin, which causes it to rise. Polarity exists at every level of biological organization. The bloodstream, for example, is counterbalanced by the lymph stream, estrogen and other female hormones by testosterone and other male hormones, DNA by RNA, red blood cells by white blood cells, growth-enhancing genes by growth-suppressing genes, activating neurotransmitters by inhibiting neurotransmitters, collagen by elastin, sodium ions by potassium ions, and so on throughout the body.

Polarities also exist in movement and function. Walking, for example, involves simultaneous up and down, forward and backward, and left and right motions. As one leg is lifted up, the other is pushed down. As one leg moves forward, the opposite arm moves backward, and so on in a series of alternating movements. In any action, certain parts of the body will be engaged in active movement, while others remain relatively still; certain parts lead, while others follow; certain muscles expand, while others contract. Periods of active movement alternate with periods of rest.

Moment to moment, we breathe in and breathe out, as the movements of the heart, lungs, and digestive organs alternate between expansion and contraction, activation and inhibition. In the morning we get up, and at night we lie down. When we speak, our voice alternates between high and low tones, rapid and slow speech, and periods of sound and silence. When we write, our hand moves up and down, we press the pen to the paper and then relax it, we begin sentences and then complete them, and move from left to right across the page. One hand holds the pen, the other supports the paper.

The rhythms of daily life—waking and sleeping, appetite and fullness, movement and rest—are animated by polarity, as are relationships between people. Some people are male, others female, some are large, others small, some are thin, others heavy, some are fair skinned, others have dark skin. Some people are intellectual, others physical, some are blonde, others brunette, some are born in the spring, others in the fall. Polarities provide the basis for comparisons between people, and underlie the relationship between self and other, I and the universe, and humanity and nature. They are at the root of all perception and evaluation. All things are composed of multiple polarities, and polarities define the relationships between all things. Reality is a unified field of countless interrelationships, all of which are defined and governed by polarity. Polarity is the one common factor unifying all of existence.

Alpha and Omega, Yin and Yang

If we consider the complex field polarities existing in ourselves and the world around us, we notice certain correspondences between them. These correspondences make it possible to categorize them in a consistent manner. Using our environment on earth as a frame of reference, let us evaluate several of the polarities cited above. We can begin with the polarity between up and down and horizontal and vertical. Movement in an upward direction means movement away from the earth, while downward movement implies movement toward the earth. (The distinction between up and down exists only in relation to physical bodies, such as stars and planets. There is no "up" or "down" in interstellar space.) If something has a predominantly vertical form, a greater portion of its mass extends upward away from the earth, while if something has a primarily horizontal form, a greater portion of its mass lies closer to the earth. Therefore, upward movement gives rise to vertical forms, while downward movement gives rise to horizontal forms.

If we view the earth from a distance, we see that the center of the earth corresponds to the inside, while the surface or periphery corresponds to the outside. In effect, downward movement means movement in an inward direction toward the center of the earth, while upward movement implies movement in an outward direction away from the center and toward the periphery. Thus we can link these pairs of opposites as follows:

upward movement (up)	downward movement (down)
vertical	horizontal
outward movement	inward movement
periphery (outside)	center (inside)

When something expands, it increases in size, and when it contracts, it becomes smaller. Largeness is a property of expansion, and smallness a property of contraction. If we relate these attributes to position, expanding force tends to push things toward the outside or periphery, while contracting force causes things to gather toward the center. Upward movement is actually outward or expanding motion away from the earth, while downward movement is actually a form of contracting motion toward the earth. Largeness and expansion are therefore consistent with the characteristics in the left-hand column, while smallness and contraction are consistent with those in the right-hand column. If we add these new attributes to our list, our classification is as follows (for convenience, we will label the attributes on the left "alpha" and those on the right "omega," using the Greek terms that denote polarity):

Alpha	**Omega**
upward movement (up)	downward movement (down)
vertical	horizontal
outward movement	inward movement
periphery (outside)	center (inside)
large	small
expansion	contraction

Now that expansion and contraction have been added to our list, it is much easier to classify a variety of other complementary attributes in either of these categories. When things absorb water, for example, they expand and become larger, and when they dry out, they contract and shrink. Therefore, wetness can be included in the alpha column, and dryness in the omega column. As things expand, they become lighter and less dense, and when they contract, they become increasingly dense and heavy. Density and heaviness can thus be grouped with the qualities under omega, while lightness can be classified under alpha. Because solids are generally dense and heavy in comparison to liquids or gases, we would classify them under omega. Liquids and gases are light and diffuse, and are thus classified under alpha.

Heat is a property of contracting force or movement, while cold is a property of expansion. Space, which is infinitely expanded, is cold, while heat is a product of condensed material forms such as stars and planets. Space is also dark. Brightness is a characteristic of the condensed points known as stars. Therefore, heat and brightness can be classified under omega, while coldness and darkness match the characteristics under alpha.

All polarities can be classified as such into two categories. The multiple polarities that comprise reality are actually nothing but varied appearances of two primary forces. Physical attributes such as temperature, size, weight, structure, form, position, and wavelength yield numerous complementary tendencies that display a stronger tendency either toward expansive force, or toward contractive force. Thousands of years ago in China, these primary forces were given the names yin and yang. The term yin refers to the primary force of expansion (centrifugal force) found throughout the universe, and corresponds to the attributes listed above in the alpha column. The term yang refers to the primary force of contraction (centripetal force) found throughout the universe, and corresponds to the attributes listed under omega. Although the terms yin and yang were first used in China, the understanding they represent is not particularly Oriental. An understanding of complementary polarity can be found in cultures throughout the world. In the table below, we classify a va-

Examples of Yin and Yang

	YIN	YANG
Attribute	Centrifugal force	Centripetal force
Tendency	Expansion	Contraction
Function	Diffusion	Fusion
	Dispersion	Assimilation
	Separation	Gathering
	Decomposition	Organization
Movement	More inactive, slower	More active, faster
Vibration	Shorter wave and higher frequency	Longer wave and lower frequency
Direction	Ascent and vertical	Descent and horizontal
Position	Outward, peripheral	Inward and central
Weight	Lighter	Heavier
Temperature	Colder	Hotter
Light	Darker	Brighter
Humidity	Wetter	Drier
Density	Thinner	Thicker
Size	Larger	Smaller
Shape	More expansive, fragile	More contractive, harder
Form	Longer	Shorter
Texture	Softer	Harder
Atomic particle	Electron	Proton
Elements	N, O, P, Ca, etc.	H, C, Na, As, Mg, etc.
Environment		
Climatic effects	Tropical climate	Colder climate
Biological	More vegetable quality	More animal quality
Sex	Female	Male
Organ structure	More hollow, expansive	Compacted, condensed
Nerves	More peripheral, orthosympathetic	More central, parasympathetic
Attitude, emotion	More gentle, negative, defensive	More active, positive, aggressive
Work	More psychological, mental	More physical, social
Consciousness	More universal	More specific
Mental function	Dealing more with the future	Dealing more with the past
Culture	More spiritually oriented	More materially oriented
Dimension	Space	Time

riety of complementary attributes into yin and yang. There are many ways to classify things into complementary categories, and this chart represents only one way based on the definition of yin and yang established above. Yin and yang are not absolute, if anything, they are absolutely relative. All things are composed of both energies, and nothing is exclusively yin or yang. Things are not yin or yang of themselves, but only in relation to other things

Yin and yang can also be expressed in terms of *heaven's* and *earth's forces.* Heaven is yin or expanded, while the earth is relatively tiny, compact, and yang. However, even though its form is yin, the universe generates movement in the form of contracting spirals, similar to the way that cold (also yin) causes things to contract. Contracting energy spirals inward and becomes progressively more condensed. As these spirals make the transition from energy to matter, they give rise to preatomic particles and atoms, creating a countless number of stars, planets, and other material objects, each of which is tiny and contracted in comparison to the surrounding universe. Heaven's energy appears on our planet as a contractive, centripetal, or downward force (yang). Because the earth continuously rotates, it gives off a stream of expansive, centrifugal, or upward force (yin).

The classification of heaven's force as yang and earth's force as yin is consistent with that found in *The Yellow Emperor's Classic of Internal Medicine.* This ancient Chinese classic, originally known as the *Nei-Ching*, was composed thousands of years ago and is believed to be one of the oldest medical texts in existence. It is attributed to the Yellow Emperor, or Ko-Tei, the last of three legendary emperors credited with establishing the foundations of Chinese philosophy and medicine. In it the sky or heaven is classified as yang, while the earth is classified as yin. The same classification appears in the *I Ching*, or *Book of Changes*, and is based on the energetic functions of heaven and earth described above. However, if we classify heaven and earth according to their physical nature, our classification is exactly opposite. Heaven is structurally large or expanded (yin), while the earth is tiny and compact (yang). As we can see, yin and yang are interchangeable. How we classify things depends on which criteria we use as the basis for our classification.

HUMAN CHARACTERISTICS
ACCORDING TO YIN AND YANG

	Yin	Yang
Sex	Female	Male
Climate of origin	Warmer, more equatorial	Colder, more northern or temperate
Diet	Based on plant foods	Based on animal foods
Body type	Tall and thin	Short and stocky
Orientation	Aesthetic or contemplative	Theoretic or active
Living Place	South or West	North or East
Facial shape	Longer and thinner	Square or round
Season of birth	Autumn or winter	Spring or summer
Hair color	Darker	Lighter
Thinking	Right brain	Left brain
Personality type	Type B (calm)	Type A (aggressive)
Attitude	Cooperative	Competitive
View of life	More spiritual and long-term	More materialistic and short-term
Technology	Low-tech	High-tech
Environment	Country	City
Pace	Slower and more relaxed	More rapid and stressful
Response	Adaptation	Modification
Politics	More liberal and progressive	More conservative

As we see in the table above, human characteristics can be classified according to yin and yang. These classifications are not absolute. A variety of individual differences exist within each of these general categories. For example, on the whole, people living in northern regions are yang in comparison to people in the tropics, due to the effects of climate and diet. Some people who live in the north, for example, are yang due to a high intake of animal foods, while others are yin because of eating plenty of fruits and vegetables. Some have yang Type A personalities, others are yin Type Bs. Some are tall and thin, others short and stocky, and some are male, others female. Some are born in the spring and summer (yang) while others are born in the fall and winter (yin). A person who eats plenty of animal food while performing hard physical labor would probably be more yang than someone who is vegetarian and who does office work, regardless of whether he lives in the north or south. A person who is yang according to one set of characteristics may be yin according to others. Therefore, a wide variety of factors need to be taken into consideration when determining whether someone is *on the whole* yin or yang.

Polarity within Polarity

Each set of polarities found in nature contains numerous subpolarities. Let us turn to the human body as an example of the principle of polarity within polarity. On the whole, the upper regions of the body are yin in relation to the lower regions. Yet each region is made up of both soft and hard parts, peripheral and central regions, expanded and contracted organs, and bioenergetic and biochemical functions. At the same time, two complementary streams of body fluid—the yang bloodstream and the yin lymph stream— run through both regions. Numerous subpolarities exist within any of these sets of polarities. If we take the bloodstream as an example, we find polarity existing between the formed elements, which are yang or solid, and the more yin liquid or plasma. Among the formed elements, polarity exists between red blood cells, which are yang or compact, and white blood cells, which are yin or expanded. Because red blood cells are far more numerous than white blood cells, the bloodstream is on the whole yang in relation to the clear lymph stream.

Red blood cells are composed of yin and yang factors. Each

cell contains a yin cell membrane and a yang cell body, and is composed of hemoglobin, a yang protein containing iron, and yin phospholipids. (Hemoglobin comprises 60 to 80 percent of the total solids of the cell; therefore, red blood cells are on the whole more yang.) Hemoglobin is itself composed of a yang iron-containing portion (hematin), and a yin simple protein (globin). Moreover, red blood cells continuously change polarity as they circulate from the central regions of the body out to the periphery and back again. When red blood cells become more yang, they bind with oxygen, a yin element. When they reverse polarity, they discharge oxygen and bind with carbon dioxide, a more yang compound.

The body's invisible, bioenergetic functions are yin in comparison to its physical, biochemical ones. Yet, among the meridians and chakras that comprise the body's energy system, certain ones are yin, others yang. (The chakras and meridians are discussed in detail in the following chapter.) The upper chakras, for example, are generally yin in relation to those in the lower body, while the meridians divide into those with an active energy flow (yang), and those with less active energy (yin). Moreover, all of the body's structures, both physical and energetic, are constantly in motion and these motions alternate between activation and inhibition, expansion and contraction, discharging and taking in.

EXAMPLES OF YIN AND YANG IN HUMAN STRUCTURE AND FUNCTION

STRUCTURES

More Yin	More Yang
Upper body	Lower body
Right side	Left side
Front	Back
Outside (periphery)	Inside (center)
Soft parts	Hard parts
Expanded parts	Contracted parts
Digestive system	Nervous system
Lymph stream	Bloodstream

White blood cells	Red blood cells
B-cells	T-cells
Suppressor T-cells	Helper T-cells
Anti-insulin	Insulin
Head hair	Body hair
Growth enhancing genes	Growth suppressing genes
Cell membranes	Cell nucleus
Elastin	Collagen
Estrogen	Testosterone
Inhibiting neurotransmitters	Activating neurotransmitters
RNA	DNA
Potassium ions	Sodium ions
Hollow organs	Solid organs

FUNCTIONS

Bioenergetic	Biochemical
Breathing in	Breathing out
Inhibition	Activation
Dilation	Contraction
Hydration	Dehydration
Discharging	Taking in
Divergence	Convergence
Relaxation	Tension
Decay	Genesis
Response	Stimulus
Oxygenation	Deoxygenation
Catabolism	Anabolism
Ascending movement	Descending movement
Mental activities	Physical activities
Slower movement	Rapid movement

Yin and yang, or the forces of expansion and contraction, exist at every level of life, from the macrocosmic to the microcosmic, within our outer and inner environments. Each person exists as a yang, contracted center within the yin, expanded environment of the earth. However, the earth itself is part of a much larger unit, the solar system, and is yang or compact in relation to this expanded environment. The solar system in turn, is tiny and compact in relation to the Milky Way galaxy of which it is a part. And, as large as it is, the galaxy is actually a compact spiral existing within the much larger environment of the universe as a whole.

Our internal environment is structured in a similar way. The organs, for example, exist as compact units (yang) within the more expanded environment of the body as a whole (yin). Each organ, in turn, provides the expanded environment for billions of compact units known as cells. Each cell, in turn, serves as the expanded environment for the condensed nucleus, while the nucleus serves as the expanded environment for tiny strands of DNA and RNA. Each strand of DNA forms the macrocosmic environment for individual molecules of protein and carbohydrate, and these provide an expanded environment for individual atoms. Atoms, which are composed largely of empty space, provide the yin, expanded environments within which preatomic particles, such as protons and electrons, exist.

Opposites Attract

Yin and yang, or complementary opposites, are not static, but dynamically changing. Everything in the universe is constantly in motion and constantly changing. Motion and change are governed by the attraction of opposites. Mutual attraction occurs everywhere, at all levels of life, and is the invisible force that drives the endless cycles of change that govern all things.

Atoms are formed by the strong attraction between positively charged protons and negatively charged electrons. A similar attraction causes atoms to combine and form molecules. Common table salt offers a good example of this principle. On the whole, sodium is a yang or contractive element, while chlorine is yin or expansive. They are strongly polarized, and therefore strongly attracted. When they combine, sodium atoms become more yang by giving up an electron to an atom of chlorine, causing the chlorine atom to become more yin. The sodium atoms then take on a positive charge, while the chlorine atoms become negatively charged. These oppositely charged atoms, or ions, bond with tremendous force, forming highly stable molecules of salt.

In each molecule of water, two atoms of hydrogen (yang) share electrons with an atom of oxygen (yin). These strongly polarized molecules link up with other molecules when the positively charged hydrogen nuclei of one molecule attract and link up with the negatively charged, peripheral electrons in the oxygen atom of a neighboring molecule. These so-called hydrogen bonds are very strong and are responsible for the tight cohesiveness of water.

DNA, the basic building block of life, is formed through the bonding and building up of basic organic compounds that occur because of mutual attraction. DNA is constructed of four nucleotide bases: adenosine, thymidine, guanine, and cytosine. Just like the positive and negative poles of a magnet, these four bases bond into pairs because of electromagnetic attraction. Thymidine is especially complementary to adenosine, and always pairs with it. Guanine is strongly polarized with cytosine, and always links up with it. Each coiled strand of DNA is held together by hydrogen bonds existing between the bases.

Hormones secreted by the endocrine glands circulate freely throughout the bloodstream, yet only affect specific "target" organs. These effects are due to the attraction of opposites. The attraction between hormone and receptor is highly specific: the molecules of a particular hormone match receptors on the cells of its "target" organ in the way that a key fits a lock. If a hormone does not match a particular receptor, it will continue circulating until it finds the receptor that complements it most perfectly. Hormones are either yin or yang, activating or inhibiting. A yang hormone, such as adrenalin, will bind only with the yin receptors that specifically match it.

Most viruses, including those associated with colds and flu, are yin in comparison to the cells of the body. The cells of the body are yang—dense and compact—and so the virus is strongly attracted to the body's cells. The attraction is so strong that the virus can penetrate the outer wall of the cell and proceed directly to its most yang region: the nucleus and the DNA within the nucleus. Once the virus enters the nucleus, it fuses with the DNA of the cell and, in a dramatic example of yang changing into yin, uses the cell's DNA to rapidly produce new viruses. The cell then disintegrates and bursts, releasing new viruses that are attracted to other cells, where this process is repeated.

The immune response acts as a buffer between the external and internal environments, and blocks the attraction between viruses and cells. The immune response is based on the huge polarity existing between "self" and "non-self." Because of this polarity, foreign substances attract the specialized white blood cells that are part of the immune response. The immune response is flexible and specific. A yin antigen, such as a virus, triggers a variety of yang responses that perfectly match and neutralize it, while a yang antigen, such as a bacteria (on the whole, bacteria are more yang than viruses) elicits a variety of yin responses that counterbalance it. In a typical immune response, a virus will attract specialized white blood cells known as *macrophages*. These yang, active cells neutralize the virus by engulfing or "eating" it. Macrophages in turn attract a type of white blood cell known as *granulocytes*. These cells release a yin substance known as *histamine* that causes openings to form in the walls of the blood vessels, thus allowing lymphocytes and other white blood cells to enter the area and creating a barrier to the spread of the virus.

At the next level of immune response, macrophages carry viruses to the thymus gland, where in a process known as *antigen recognition*, sensitive lymphocytes read its characteristics. A variety of specialized cells are involved in this process, and they can be divided into two general categories: yin B-cells, and yang T-cells. T-cells further differentiate into helper T-cells that turn on the immune response (yang), and suppressor T-cells that shut it off (yin).

The helper T-cells stimulate the B-cells to secrete antibodies, natural substances that are opposite to the virus but that match it in the way that hormones specifically match the receptors on cells. Because the virus and antibody are specifically matched, they are strongly attracted to each other. After being secreted by B-cells, antibodies coat the virus, covering its receptors and blocking its attraction to the body's cells. Antibodies do this by interfering with the polarity that exists between the virus and the body's cells. By *yangizing* the virus, they make it less strongly attracted to the body's cells (yang). Once a virus has been neutralized in this manner, it attracts strong yin enzymes, similar to digestive enzymes, that dissolve it. (This process is known as complement activity.) Then, in a parallel process, other T-cells, known as *effector cells*, neutralize cells that have been penetrated by the virus. These cells have been *yinnized* by the virus and, as a result, attract these strongly yang T-cells.

Natural immunity is animated by the polarity between self and non-self, antigen and antibody, T-cells and B-cells, helper cells and suppressor cells. The immune response is not a process of war or battle, but a process of natural harmony. Viruses and other antigens are not "enemies" or "invaders," but a natural part of our environment. The modern notion of "cell wars," in which the immune system is described as a battlefield, is based on an incomplete understanding of the harmony of opposites found throughout nature.

Human appetites are based on the attraction of opposites. When we are hungry, we are attracted to food; when active, we are attracted to rest; when lonely, we are attracted to companionship; when stressed, we are attracted to relaxation; and when overworked, we are attracted to leisure. Relationships between the sexes are a particularly dynamic expression of this principle. Men and women have opposite energies; men receive a stronger charge of heaven's downward force, and women, a stronger charge of earth's rising energy. The attraction between heaven's force (yang) and earth's force (yin) is the invisible, driving force behind love and sexuality. To quote Tielhard de Chardin:

> If there were no internal propensity to unite, even at a prodigiously rudimentary level—indeed in the molecule itself—it would be physically impossible for love to appear higher up.

Human reproductive cells—the egg and sperm—are strongly polarized and therefore strongly attracted. Even though women are on the whole more yin than men, the human ovum is concentrated and strongly yang. Sperm are created through a process of differentiation and are strongly yin. (Only one egg is released at a time; several hundred million sperm are discharged in one ejaculation.) The egg and sperm are so strongly polarized that their union results in more than just a simple combination, in which two opposites join but retain their separate identities. The union of egg and sperm results in a complete fusion in which both lose their individual identities and merge into an entirely new being that blends the qualities of both into one.

The attraction of opposites always produces dramatic results. When egg and sperm unite, they begin a dramatic new process that culminates in the appearance of a new human being. When a man and a woman unite in love, they create a unity that transcends the individuality of each. When oxygen combines with hydrogen, these two elements create a new substance—water—that bears little resemblance to the two invisible gases that create it. When yin and yang unite, yin becomes less yin and yang becomes less yang. The degree of attraction depends on the degree of polarity. The more strongly polarized things are, the more strongly they are attracted, and the more they change once they unite with their opposite.

Likes Repel

Counterbalancing the universal force of attraction is a universal force of repulsion. Just as opposites attract, likes repel. The force of attraction can be considered yang; it represents the fusion or coming together of opposites. The force of repulsion is yin; it results in the separation or coming apart of likes. Examples of repulsion abound in nature. Two positive electric charges or magnetic poles repel each other, as do two negative poles. Bright colors, which are yang, reflect sunlight, while yin dark colors absorb it. Animals, which are yang in relation to plants, breathe in or attract oxygen, a yin gas, while breathing out or repelling yang carbon dioxide. Being yin, plants perform the opposite function: they absorb carbon dioxide and repel oxygen.

In the world of subatomic particles, electrons and protons continually attract and repel one another. When two hydrogen atoms approach each other, both of their protons are attracted to the electrons of the other. An electrochemical bond is formed, creating a hydrogen molecule. However, as the two atoms approach one another, the forces of repulsion also come into play. Both electrons repel each other, as do the protons, and this tends to push the two atoms apart. Because electrons are mobile, they tend to occupy positions as far away from each other, and as close to both protons, as possible. This allows the forces of attraction to prevail over those of repulsion, and the two atoms bond and form a molecule.

The movement of heat follows the pattern of attraction and repulsion. Heat is repelled by itself: it flows from hotter objects to colder ones. Moreover, substances that are yang have a greater resistance to heat (also yang) than more yin ones. As a result, metals, which are solid and yang, have much higher melting temperatures than more yin liquids or gases.

The immune response involves forces of repulsion and forces of attraction. The responses of the immune system are triggered by the polarity that exists between self and non-self. Immune cells are attracted to substances they determine to be "non-self," and their responses are aimed at neutralizing the polarity these substances have with the cells of the body. When antibodies coat a virus, for example, they reverse the polarity of its receptor mechanisms, causing them to become more yang. As a result, rather than being attracted to the body's cells, the virus is now repelled by the body's cells. The reversal of polarity renders the virus inactive by interfering with its ability to bind with cells. Normally, the immune response stops once foreign substances, such as virus or bacteria, have been neutralized and discharged from the body. Cells of the immune system do not react to the cells of the body. Immune cells and body cells are similar in that they are both "self," and are therefore repelled by one another.

However, this healthy repulsion can change into unhealthy attraction if either the immune or body cells start to change. If either variety of cells degenerates due to extreme dietary imbalances, they may start to attract one another, triggering an immune response. This process underlies so-called autoimmune diseases such as rheumatoid arthritis and lupus erythematosus.

The closer two oppositely charged objects are to each other, the more strongly attracted they are. The closer two similarly charged objects are to each other, the more strongly repelled they are. Attraction and repulsion are also influenced by time. When any two opposites bond with each other, they both start to change. They become more like each other and less strongly attracted. When men and women marry, for example, the husband tends to become more yin, more domestic, while the wife becomes more yang, or assertive. The strong polarity that existed to bring the two together becomes more equalized. In the case of sex, it is impossible to continue sex indefinitely; there must be a period of separation so that a man can regain his masculinity and a woman her femininity. Then the cycle of attraction can be repeated. Parents and children are strongly attracted to each other because of the strong polarity existing between them, and are united by bonds of love and affection. However, as children grow into adults, this attraction becomes less strong and can change into repulsion. That is why grown children leave home and seek an independent life in the outside world.

As we know from daily life, whenever we are attracted to something, we are at the same time being repelled (or less attracted) by something else. Whatever it is we seek, be it food, health, rest, companionship, adventure, or success, is making balance with our present condition. We are attracted to what we lack, and are repelled by what we have. When we are hungry, we eat, and when we are full, we stop eating. If we are extremely active, we are attracted to rest. After a period of relaxation, we seek new activity. Attraction and repulsion continuously alternate with one another, creating perpetual cycles of movement and change. Yin continuously changes into yang, and yang changes into yin. The alternation of opposites can be found everywhere, from the life cycle of cells to the life cycle of galaxies, and from the rhythm of the tides to the rhythm of the heart. Understanding the universal pattern of change is essential if we wish to penetrate the source of health and healing.

Cycles of Energy

At any given moment, water exists in a variety of completely different forms in the environment. Think of the placid stillness of a pond and compare that to the active rush of water down a mountain stream. Then observe ice crystals, and compare them to the invisible molecules of water vapor in the air. In all of these appearances, we are still talking about the same substance—water. The many forms of water are a perfect example of the diversity that arises from unity.

Water in its various forms is not static. It is constantly moving and changing form. Water is like a phantom that appears and disappears. One moment you see it, and in the next, you do not. In one incarnation, it may appear calm and peaceful, and in the next, turbulent and powerful.

In all of its forms and changes, water obeys the laws of yin and yang. It continually cycles back and forth between expansion and contraction. Its cyclic movements are a perfect example of the endless cycles that govern all things. Most of the water on earth exists in a yang or condensed form in the ocean. A small percentage exists as fresh water, most of which is locked into glaciers and polar ice caps in the form of ice. In its more yin forms, water exists as invisible water vapor that rises into the atmosphere, and as clouds above the earth's surface. Here it condenses and eventually falls as rain or other forms of precipitation in a continuous cycle.

The cycling of elements through the biosphere is also governed by yin and yang. The carbon and nitrogen cycles, both of which are vital to life, offer good examples. In their more yin forms, these elements exist as gases—atmospheric carbon dioxide and atmospheric nitrogen—and are converted by living organisms into more yang forms. (This process is known as "fixing.") Plants fix carbon dioxide through the process of photosynthesis. Once fixed, carbon goes in several different directions before returning to a gaseous state. Fixed carbon is used to form the structure of the plant, and takes the form of cellulose, proteins, and lipids, and some is broken down to supply energy for cellular activities. Some carbon is stored for long periods in the form of wood, coal, and oil, and some is eventually burned and returned to the atmosphere. Some organic carbon is eaten by animals and people and broken down through the process of digestion, and discharged into the atmosphere through respiration.

Gaseous nitrogen forms about 70 percent of the earth's atmosphere. Bacteria, fungi, and algae fix nitrogen in the form of nitrite, and this is in turn provided to plants and used for their growth and development. These symbiotic bacteria live within the root systems of plants and receive nutrients from the plant tissues. Symbiotic relationships, which occur everywhere in nature, are an example of the attraction and harmony of opposites. Bacteria and plants complement and benefit each other. Nitrate, a waste product of bacteria, serves as a nutrient source for plants. Nitrogen is used by the plant—in the form of nitrate—to form amino acids, proteins, nucleic acids, and other compounds. When plants die, bacteria decompose these compounds back into atmospheric nitrogen. When animals or humans eat plants, they discharge nitrogen compounds through excretion. Through a series of biochemical processes, bacteria convert these organic residues back into atmospheric nitrogen, and thus the cycle begins again.

In each of these cycles, there is a complete and continuous movement in a circular fashion, in which two opposite yet complementary movements occur. Carbon, nitrogen, and water continuously cycle back and forth between contraction and expansion, downward and upward movement, solidification and diffusion. This alternating rhythm of yin and yang is found everywhere; from the waxing and waning of the moon to the changing of the seasons and cycle of day and night, and represents the fundamental pattern of movement itself.

The basic polarity that gives rise to these alternating rhythms also creates numerous subpolarities. For example, the movement of the earth around the sun gives rise to two primary divisions—winter, which is cold, dark, and yin, and summer, which is bright, hot, and yang. They represent the main poles in the repeating cycle of the seasons. Each of these movements further subdivides so that four seasons are produced. Spring represents the early form of summer, and so we classify it as small yang, while autumn represents the early stage of winter, or small yin. Small yang eventually develops into large yang, and small yin changes into large yin.

Moreover, each of the four seasons divides further into an early and late stage, such as early summer and late summer. These subdivisions yield eight clearly defined stages of change or transformation. The cycle of the seasons is but one example of the way all movements alternate between yin and yang. The cycle of day and night offers another example. The greatest polarity in the daily cycle is that between night (large yin) and day (large yang). Morning represents the early stage of day and corresponds to small yang, and evening, the early stage of night, to small yin. These opposite poles subdivide into early and late stages, yielding eight defined stages in the daily cycle.

In both of these cycles, one basic movement (e.g., the revolution of the earth around the sun or the rotation of the earth on its axis) gives rise to a recurring cycle based on the alternation of two opposite states. These opposites further divide into two, and each of these stages also divides into two. The process of subdivision is actually endless and arises because of the basic waving pattern of all motion in the universe. All things pass through these stages in their evolution and development. The understanding of these recurring cycles is at the heart of Oriental and other traditional cosmologies, including Buddhism and the *I Ching.* The *I Ching* is based on a recurring cycle of sixty-four stages of change. Each stage is represented by a symbol, or hexagram, made up of six lines, with unbroken lines representing yang force or movement, and broken lines representing yin activity.

Ancient thinkers in the West, including Pythagoras, Aristotle, and Plato, were aware of the cyclic movements governing nature. They believed that these natural cycles are without beginning or end. Modern science has replaced this circular, cyclic view of time with the concept of time as a linear, or straight line motion. Scientists have the tendency to think that the universe began at some fixed point, such as the "big bang," rather than seeing the process of creation, destruction, and new creation as the expression of an eternal cycle. In reality, the flow of time is neither circular nor linear. Time unfolds in the form of a spiral. The spiral model explains why things are always new and fresh, yet change according to a repeating pattern.

The Five Energies

Cycles of change can be understood in terms of five recurring stages. This cycle, known as the five transformations, or *Go-Gyo*, lies at the heart of Oriental medicine, and is related to the ancient healing system of India, and to the medical philosophy of Hippocrates. It is a fundamental principle of holistic healing. This cycle describes the movement of energy through five progressive states. It is basically a more elaborate way of expressing the alternation between expansion and contraction, or yin and yang, found throughout nature. The cycle describes the dynamic movement of energy, not the interrelationship of static "elements." Referring to it as the "five element theory" is incorrect.

The world of matter, for example, is governed by cycles in which substances move back and forth between a yang or condensed phase and a yin, or expanded one. In its most diffused or energetic state, matter decomposes into its constituent parts. When heat is applied, the forces that hold molecules together break down. If more heat is applied, molecules break down into individual atoms, and if an even greater amount of heat is applied, atoms decompose into preatomic particles, such as when hydrogen breaks down into free electrons and protons. This energized state of matter is known as plasma, and is created when a gas is heated to a high temperature. In traditional Oriental cosmology, this diffused and energized state is referred to as *Ka-Sei*, or fire nature.

Upon reaching this diffused state, a yang process of solidification or condensation takes over and causes atomic particles to condense into atoms, and atoms to bond with each other to form molecules. In this process, known traditionally as *Do-Sei*, or soil nature, molecular bonding forces become stronger, and matter assumes a definite form.

In its least energetic state, matter exists in a solid form. Solids exist in two types: yin amorphous solids, such as glass, which display many of the properties of a viscous liquid, and yang crystalline solids. In solid matter, the forces of molecular bonding are strong enough to lock the atoms and molecules of a substance into rigid alignment. In contrast to plasmas, which are composed of diffused, energetic, and freely moving ions, the atoms and molecules in a crystal are densely packed and have a limited range of motion. Appropriately enough, ancient people referred to this yang, condensed state as *Kin-Sei*, or metal nature.

When a solid is exposed to energy, especially heat, its atoms and molecules begin to absorb energy and vibrate rapidly. The solid melts and changes into a liquid. The molecules of a liquid move more actively than do those of a solid, and have a relatively freer range of motion, yet are held together by strong forces of molecular bonding. In traditional cosmology, this state of change is referred to as *Sui-Sei*, or water nature.

If the molecules of a liquid are further energized, for example, through a rise in temperature, the forces of molecular attraction can be overcome, causing the substance to decompose. Molecules enter a condition of rapid and random motion, and the resulting state is known as a gas. In traditional cosmology, this actively expanding stage is referred to as *Moku-Sei*, or tree nature.

These five stages are found throughout nature and can be summarized as (1) ascending, rapidly expanding energy, or tree nature; (2) very expanded, activated free energy, or fire nature; (3) gathering, condensing, downward and inward moving energy, or soil nature; (4) fully consolidated, materialized energy or

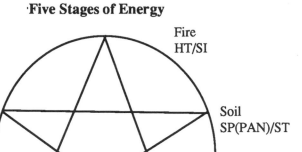

·Five Stages of Energy

metal nature; and (5) slowly dissolving, floating energy on the borderline between strong condensation and strong expansion, or water nature.

Organs and the Five Energies

The bodily organs can be divided into two general categories. The organs are structured in pairs, one being yin and the other yang. The lungs and large intestine form an organ pair. The lungs are positioned in the upper body; the large intestine in the lower region. The lungs are packed with air sacs and blood vessels, and have a dense, compact structure, while the large intestine is a long, hollow tube. The lungs are structurally yang, and thus process gas (yin), while the structurally yin large intestine processes digested solids and liquids (yang). The degree of complementarity between these organs is very great.

The heart and small intestine also function as a pair. Their complementarity can be seen in their position—the heart in the upper body, and the small intestine in the lower—and in their structure—the heart is a compact muscle and the small intestine, an extended hollow tube. The structurally yang heart distributes blood throughout the body, while the structurally yin small intestine is the site in which nutrients are absorbed into the bloodstream for eventual distribution to all of the body's cells.

The kidneys and bladder comprise another complementary pair. The kidneys are solid and compact, and the bladder is hollow and expanded. The structurally yang kidneys are located toward the back of the body, while the structurally yin bladder is located toward the front.

The spleen and pancreas share the same blood and energy streams and in Oriental medicine, were considered as the differentiation of one meridian or energy system. They are complementary to the stomach. The spleen and pancreas both have a dense, compact structure (yang), and the stomach has a yin, hollow and expanded structure.

The liver and gallbladder are opposite in structure—the liver being compact and yang, and the gallbladder taking the form of a yin hollow sac. The degree of complementarity between these organs is much less than that of the lungs and large intestine, heart and small intestine, and kidneys and bladder.

Each of the organ pairs corresponds to one of the stages of the five transformations. The liver and gallbladder are manifestations of tree energy; the heart and small intestine, fire energy; the spleen, pancreas, and stomach, soil energy; the lungs and large intestine, metal energy; and the kidneys and bladder, water energy. This classification can be found in *The Yellow Emperor's Classic of Internal Medicine*. However, it is important to understand why the organs are classified in this manner. The key to this is the understanding of energy. In Chapter 7, we explain why the organs are classified this way. Before reading this chapter, however, please try to discover on your own why the organs have this particular classification.

Cycles of Health and Sickness

All of the body's functions, including those involved in sickness and healing, can be understood according to the five transformations. We can take the common cold as an example. Colds and flu typically follow a natural course, and represent the movement of excessive energy within the body. The typical cold cycle begins with a yin, expansive and outward phase, and finishes with a yang, inward or consolidating phase. The yin phase is commonly called the acute or early stage. It usually lasts for three or four days, during which excess begins to accumulate and is discharged, primarily in an upward direction through the respiratory passages. The discharge is usually watery and loose at first, and inflammation begins and spreads throughout the mucous membranes of the nose and throat. Fever begins during this stage and the person may start to discharge through coughing.

Once the initial phase has been completed, the discharge enters a phase of consolidation and resolution. This is commonly known as the late stage of the cold. The thin, watery discharge usually becomes thicker and yellowish in color. The immune system becomes active and resists further spread of inflammation, and appetite and energy start to return. Swollen, inflamed mucous membranes gradually return to a more normal, contracted state. Coughing usually continues through this stage, and may be worse in the evening when, according to the daily cycle of energy, the lungs and large intestine are especially active.

Ultimately, the body's normal discharge processes take over and handle the elimination of remaining excess. Discharge is then accomplished through the kidneys, skin, lungs, and intestines. At that time, the cold resolves itself and the person returns to a normal condition.

The cold cycle can be divided into five general stages corresponding to the five transformations. The stages of onset and acute symptoms represent more yin, or outward phases, and correspond to tree and fire nature. The stages in which excess gathers and consolidates are more yang and correspond to soil and metal nature. The final breakup or resolution of the cold corresponds to the stage of water nature.

Degenerative conditions can also be charted according to the five transformations. Several years ago I spoke with a man who had cancer. Two years before he had felt a strange sensation in the abdomen and went to a hospital. An examination revealed cancer of the colon, and an operation was performed in which part of the colon was removed. He was also given chemotherapy. For a while it appeared that the cancer had been controlled, so he returned to work.

However, after one year he started to feel pressure in the lower abdomen. An examination revealed that his prostate gland had become enlarged. Upon further examination, it was discovered that his prostate was cancerous. The prostate consists of seven layers, and in his case, five were cancerous. During the examination, the doctors noticed that he had a condition that appeared to be jaundice. None of the doctors could explain why the cancer had spread from the colon to the prostate.

According to the five transformations, the colon represents metal energy. From metal, the cycle of energy changes to the stage of water. The kidneys and bladder are classified as water organs. The prostate is closely related to the kidneys and bladder, and also represents water energy. In this case, the cancer was spreading in accord with the flow of energy through the five transformations, originating in the colon (metal) and then appearing in the prostate (water).

According to this process, in which part of the body would the cancer appear next? It would appear in the organs that correspond to tree energy, or in other words, the liver or gallbladder. The observation that jaundice was developing confirmed that problems were indeed starting in these organs. As I point out in *The Cancer-Prevention Diet* (New York: St. Martin's Press, 1983), there are two broad categories of cancer—one caused by the excessive intake of extreme yang foods such as meat, eggs, chicken, cheese, and other animal products, and the other by the excessive intake of extreme yin foods including refined sugar, chemicals, ice cream, chocolate, and processed foods. The cycle of the five transformations can help us understand the cause of this cancer. The overall movement of energy in this case is toward yin. Which region of the colon is most yin—the ascending colon, transverse colon, or descending colon? The ascending colon is most yin, since it develops in an upward direction. It was here that this man's cancer first appeared. The cancer began in an organ corresponding to metal energy, and then spread toward water and tree energy, following the movement of energy in a yin, upward direction.

Why did the cancer begin at the stage of metal energy? There are two broad categories of food—yin and yang, or plant foods and animal foods. Which of these types causes cancer in regions of the body corresponding to metal, the most condensed or yang of the stages of transformation?

Cancers appearing in the contracted regions of the body are caused by too much yang. Since yin and yang together result in harmony, yang, compacted regions of the body can absorb a greater volume of yin than more expanded regions. For example, when someone is physically active, he can take in more water and oxygen, both of which are yin. In terms of activity, the lungs and large intestine are more yang, since they are constantly working. They both attract and process yin substances; air, in the case of the lungs, and water in the case of the large intestine.

Because of their yang natures, these organs have a low tolerance for strong yang foods. This man's cancer appeared in the large intestine, and was caused by too much animal food. However, since the cancer appeared in the yin ascending colon, and was progressing in a yin direction, dairy food, which is a yin form of animal food, was the primary cause. Milk is a yin form of dairy, while cheese is condensed or yang. This man's cancer was caused primarily from an excessive intake of milk. He had a milky complexion and he mentioned that he had consumed three or four glasses of milk per day for more than twenty years. Other dietary extremes, such as overconsumption of meat, eggs, chicken, cheese, sugar, and chemicals contributed to his problem, but his overintake of milk was the primary cause.

Supporting and Overriding Energies

If we view the complete cycle of five stages as one continuous sequence, we see that each stage naturally supports or produces the energy of the following stage: soil energy creates and supports metal energy, which in turn gives birth to and reinforces water energy. Water nature creates and nourishes tree energy, and so forth. This sequential relationship is called the *Shen cycle*, or cycle of creation. The relationship of each stage to the next is called the parent-child relationship.

The other basic relationship to consider is that of each energy stage to those stages lying at the opposite half of the cycle. When the gathering, consolidating energy of soil nature is emphasized, naturally the opposite, dissolving or dispersing energy of water nature is inhibited. When water nature energy is encouraged, the energetic, active stage of fire nature is suppressed. Fire nature energy tends to cancel out or prevent the heavily materializing energy of metal nature, and so forth. This cycle of suppression or control is called the *Ko cycle*.

In subsequent chapters, we discuss this cycle in greater depth and explain how it can be used to understand the relationship between body and mind, humanity and nature, for the purposes of healing and regeneration.

The Cycle of Twelve

Traditional people also employed a cycle of twelve to divide the hours of the day, the months, and the years. The division of the cycle of yin and yang into twelve stages formed the basis for ancient cosmologies and healing systems in both East and West, and gave rise to the development of calendars, of which our modern calendar is a descendant. The twelve divisions correspond to the flow of electromagnetic energy, or Ki, in the earth's atmosphere and through the body during the course of a day, month, or year. The twelve-year cycle corresponds to the approximately twelve-year revolution of Jupiter around the sun and to the recurring cycle of sunspot peaks and lows. Each of these twelve divisions also corresponds to one of the twelve constellations of the zodiac. In all, there are fourteen meridians in our body that run on the surface of the skin; two, known as the governing and conception vessels, come from the original forces of heaven and earth. The remaining twelve correspond to the twelve constellations as follows:

Meridian	Constellation
Lung	Aires
Large Intestine	Taurus
Stomach	Gemini
Spleen	Cancer
Heart	Leo
Small Intestine	Virgo
Bladder	Libra
Kidney	Scorpio
Heart Governor	Sagittarius
Triple Heater	Capricorn
Gallbladder	Aquarius
Liver	Pisces

Two of the meridians do not correspond to organs, but to body-wide functions. The heart governor corresponds to the overall circulation of blood and other fluids throughout the body, while the triple heater represents the comprehensive function of body metabolism, including the generation of heat and energy. The correspondences between the constellations and meridians —or outer and inner environments—originates during the embryonic period. The uterus is covered by invisible energy lines that are like the ridges on a squash or pumpkin. These lines conduct a powerful charge of electromagnetic energy, or Ki. The uterus is aligned along the mother's primary channel of energy, and receives a strong charge of heaven's and earth's forces. At its center is the hara chakra, one of the seven strongly charged energy centers in the body.

There are many similarities between the invisible energy system and the body-wide network of nerve cells. Both systems begin from a vertical line that runs through the center of the body. In the case of the energy system, this central line takes the form of a primary channel that flows deep within the body from the top of the head to the sexual organs. In the nervous system, it takes the form of the brain and spinal cord. The meridians radiate outward from the primary channel, while numerous peripheral nerves branch outward from the brain and spinal cord. The meridians originate within the highly charged energy centers known as *chakras*, and differentiate until they connect with each of the body's cells. The peripheral nerves emerge from the compact vertebrae that appear along the spine, and differentiate into many tiny nerve branches. There are twelve primary meridians branching from the primary channel, and twelve pairs of cranial nerves emerge from the brain.

When a fertilized ovum implants itself in the wall of the uterus, it begins to receive a strong charge of energy from the uterine meridians. This charge creates a strong energy field around the ovum, similar to the energy field surrounding the earth. The ovum begins to grow within this powerfully charged environment. The powerful energy that charges the uterus causes the fertilized ovum to spin actively, like the earth. On the surface of the earth, the force coming down from the universe (heaven's force) is stronger than the upward force being generated by the rotation of the planet. The predominance of heaven's force causes the ovum to extend downward on either side, while earth's force pushes up at the center, creating a split in the middle that causes the cell to divide into two. When the process of division reaches a certain point, an axis shift arises, just as it does from time to time on earth. The two daughter cells then begin to spin on a new axis and receive heaven's and earth's forces from a new direction. Soon, cell division again takes place, and another axis shift occurs. This happens many, many times, as the cells divide from one to two, four, eight, and so forth, eventually creating a multicellular organism. Throughout this process, these new cells are charged by various stars and celestial phenomena, and coordinate very beautifully with the cosmos.

This mass of multiplying cells eventually begins to take on a definite embryonic form. During this time, heaven's and earth's forces directly influence this formation. The embryo also receives energy directly from the uterine ridges, or energy meridians. Since in its early stages, the embryo is still rotating, energy from the uterine meridians curves or spirals inward toward its center. In the central regions deep inside the embryo, these energies collect in dense, compact spirals, and are then discharged outward in the form of two huge streams of energy. One stream divides into two and becomes the arms, and other divides and becomes the legs.

We can see traces of the same process, for example, in the formation of a watermelon: if you halve a watermelon at the center, you can see a belt going around the periphery, spiraling in toward the inside and creating small, dense centers of energy. In the case of a watermelon, we call these *seeds*, while in the human body, we call these gathering places *organs*.

It is along the outer edge of the embryo that energy from the uterine meridians first enters the newly developing human form. This outer edge eventually becomes our back and spine. Energy gathers deep inside the embryo and from here is discharged outward. This inner region eventually becomes the front of the body, including the digestive vessels. This current begins where energy from the uterine meridians enters the developing embryo. Then it gathers toward the center and creates dense spirals, or organs, and from here is discharged, forming the arms and legs. This entire current of energy is called the *meridian system*. Organs are not separate from meridians; they are simply the most dense or physical part of this entire process. Organs and meridians are part of one flowing continuum of energy.

The twelve currents of energy enter the developing embryo from the twelve meridians in the mother's uterus. The uterine meridians, in turn, are formed by the mother's own twelve body meridians. The source of energy exists outside the body in the surrounding universe. The energy that charges the meridians originates in the twelve constellations of the zodiac. So, throughout life, the activity of the twelve meridians and organs is influenced and governed, not only by the type of food we take in and by the energy in our immediate environment, but also by the activities of the twelve constellations. That is why each meridian is particularly active at certain times of day and during certain months, according to which of the twelve constellations is most strongly influencing us at that time.

Spiral Motion

All movement in the universe occurs in the form of spirals. We can find traces of the spiral pattern in the movement of galaxies in the macrocosmic world, and in the formation of cells and preatomic particles in the microcosmic universe. The movements of daily life are reflections of this spiral pattern.

As we have seen, walking involves various complementary movements such as upward and downward, forward and backward, and expansive and contractive motion. These motions are all variations of one theme. The arms and legs are actually logarithmic spirals with seven orbits. We can see this clearly if we study their curled formation during the embryonic period. All movements occur because the various spirals of the human body are either contracted or rotated inward, or expanded or rotated outward. The arms, hands, and fingers can be curled either toward or away from the body, or rotated toward the right or left. The legs and feet also move in a similar pattern, as does the head, neck, spine, and torso. The organs and meridians take the form of energy spirals, as do each of the seven chakras, or energy centers, deep within the body.

The universe as a whole is structured as a vast logarithmic spiral. Each of us exists at the center of a huge spiral that originates within the infinite universe. In the infinite ocean of the universe, beyond time and space, infinite streams of expanding motion arise. They move in all directions at infinite speed. When lines of infinite expanding force intersect, spirals arise, like whirlpools in a stream. These spirals are formed by centripetal force and wind inward. They give birth to the world of matter, and when they reach the center, they begin to expand and eventually dissolve back into infinite expansion. Each of these spirals gives rise to a complete universe.

Spiral of Materialization

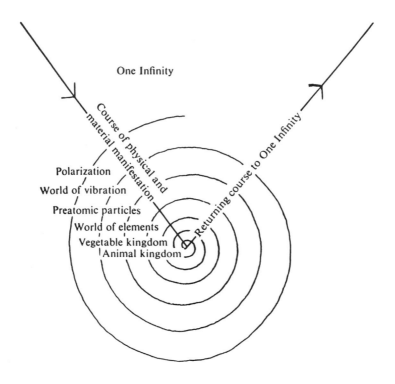

Our universe came into being because of the appearance of two complementary forces: the centripetal, materializing force that causes spirals to form, and the centrifugal, spiritual force that causes them to dissolve. These primary forces, which we refer to as yin and yang, give birth to space and time, and to the relative, ever-changing world. The primary polarization of the infinite universe creates the world of energy, or vibrations, and these travel along an incoming spiral and become condensed, giving birth to the world of matter. The condensation of energy gives rise to infinitesimally small units known as electrons, protons, and other pre-atomic particles. These condense further into elements, and on the earth and other planets throughout the universe, elements in the soil, water, and air combine with energy to create plant life. Plants in turn condense into animal life, and ultimately into human life. When we see this process of cosmic transformation from our point of view, we can say that we attract or take in the various worlds that comprise our environment in the universe. When we see it from the point of view of the universe, however, it can be said that these worlds continuously change into one another and ultimately transform themselves into human life.

Our infinitesimally small world is a condensed form of the infinitely large world. At the same time, infinity is an expanded form of the infinitesimal world. Infinity moves at absolute speed, beyond time or space. The infinitesimal world moves at relative speed and is defined by space and time, expansion and contraction, beginning and end. These worlds are not separate. One is a continuation of the other.

Infinity is the origin of this tiny, relative world, including all human beings. Infinity did not create us, but changed into us. And we will eventually return to the infinite universe. We are one with the infinite universe, and achieving this realization is actually the goal of self-healing.

Although vegetables, animals, atoms, and molecules are manifestations of infinity, in our sensory domain, we regard them as separate material things. However, their existence is fundamentally vibrational. The difference between things that exist physically, such as cells, tissues, and organs, and those existing in the form of invisible energy, such as chakras and meridians, depends on whether their speed of vibration is slow or fast, condensed or diffused. Things composed of slower, more dense vibrations we consider material. Things with a higher vibrational rate we define as mental or spiritual. The material world is the visible front that we perceive with the senses. The vibrational world is the invisible back that we perceive through intuition. They are different aspects of the same reality.

Implications for Health and Healing

The ways in which these principles can be applied to health and healing are unlimited. If we take the principle of unity in diversity as an example, we see that everyone has a different physical and mental condition, yet these differences spring from common causes. Dietary and lifestyle imbalances are the most common causes of illness today. Lifestyle imbalances are like the trunk of a tree, out of which an endless diversity of symptoms appear just like branches and leaves. Moreover, because everyone is more or less eating what we can term the "modern diet," people today share many conditions in common. The following conditions, for example, underlie over 75 percent of the serious diseases in our society.

Deposits of Fat and Mucus Practically everyone today has this problem to one degree or another. The general feeling is one of stuffiness or blockage in the face and head, instead of the normal feeling of clarity. Mucus deposits also appear in the lungs and reproductive organs. Liquid from these deposits is discharged from the nose, eyes, and lungs. It also takes the form of earwax and vaginal discharge. Deposits of fat and mucus are a primary cause of menstrual irregularity, and if the Fallopian tubes become blocked, infertility results. In men, these deposits appear in the prostate gland, causing enlargement and a decrease in sexual appetite and impotence. Mucus deposits can lead to the formation of cysts and stones deep inside the organs.

Excessive mucus causes other symptoms such as headaches, loss of memory, hay fever, allergies, stuttering, swollen glands, thyroid problems, and difficulty in breathing. Deposits of mucus and fat in the intestines interfere with the digestion and absorption of food. We usually interpret these symptoms as being different conditions, but they all stem from the same cause.

Deposits of fat and mucus are caused by the overconsumption of foods such as fruit, fruit juice, sugar, cheese, milk, animal fat, soymilk, oil, and nut butters. Eating any food in excess leads to the production of excess fat and mucus in the body. The intake of flour products, even those made from whole grain flours, will cause mucus to form if they are eaten too often. If you give floury cereal or soymilk to a baby every day, for example, the baby will become swollen and watery. Even if your diet is generally balanced, if you eat too many flour products, nut butters, fruit, or too many oily or greasy dishes, your body will produce deposits of mucus and you may not feel as clear, active, and positive as you would normally.

To see whether or not you have these deposits, check the whites of the eyes. If you see white or yellow under the bottom lid next to the eyeball, it is sign of fat and mucus in the body, especially in the reproductive organs. This is frequently a sign of vaginal discharge and enlargement of the prostate.

Intestinal Problems The condition of the intestines appears in the lips. If the lower lip is swollen or bulging, it is a sign of intestinal trouble. If the lip is bulging and soft, the person is prone to diarrhea. If it is swollen and hard, or if the lips are tight and thin, the person is prone to constipation. If there is a white color to the lips, there is not enough blood circulation in the intestines. Energy-activating treatments such as ginger compress and massage are helpful in these cases, as they stimulate circulation. Eating lightly cooked green vegetables on a daily basis helps relieve constipation.

In addition, thorough chewing and not eating for several hours before sleeping are helpful in restoring health to the digestive organs. It is important to minimize intake of baked flour products and oily or greasy dishes. Miso soup, with wakame sea vegetable and a variety of land vegetables, helps strengthen the intestines.

General Tiredness Fatigue is related to problems with the blood and circulation. A person who is tired all the time may be suffering from anemia. In order to check for this condition, touch the shoulders. If they are loose and the muscles are expanded (from excess fat and protein), there is a good possibility that the person is anemic. The shoulders and body as a whole should be firm but flexible, without a lot of excess. You can also see the nails. If they turn white when you stretch your fingers, it is a sign of anemia.

Anemia and fatigue arise when the proportion and combination of foods are unbalanced. Improper cooking and a lack of thorough chewing contribute to these conditions. If you take too much salt, liquid, or if you eat sugar or meat, for example, you will have a tendency to become tired. An optimal diet is based on about 50 percent whole grains, followed by 25 to 30 percent local vegetables, 5 to 10 percent sea vegetables and beans, and occasional supplementary foods such as low-fat white meat fish and seasonal fruit. Overeating also contributes to an overall feeling of tiredness, as does eating before sleeping. If your daily diet is balanced and if you are physically active, this condition will normally disappear.

General tiredness also results from chronic low blood sugar, or hypoglycemia. This condition is caused by the overintake of animal foods such as chicken, cheese, and eggs. Foods such as these, which contain plenty of saturated fat, make the pancreas become hard and tight. In this condition, the pancreas may not secrete enough glucagon, or anti-insulin. This hormone raises the level of sugar in the blood, and complements the function of insulin. When the blood sugar drops below normal, a person feels mentally and physically tired, and craves sugar, chocolate, or sweets in order to provide the body with a quick source of glucose. Tiredness resulting from hypoglycemia tends to be prevalent in the afternoon.

Skin Problems Discoloration of the skin is a reflection of internal imbalance. If the first section of the fingers is more red than the lower sections, it is a sign of coldness at the surface of the body due to poor circulation. Peripheral coldness is yin and is caused by eating too much fruit, salad, cold drinks, ice cream, and foods that chill the body. When your condition becomes healthy and sensitive, if you eat even one raw apple before you sleep, you will feel cold the following day. If the inside of the body is cold, it is from eating too much salt. When fat and mucus build up in the kidneys, intestines, and lungs, excess that would normally be discharged through these organs may start to come out through the skin, producing a variety of skin disorders, including acne, pimples, psoraisis, and eczema. Skin markings and growths are also a sign of the discharge of excess from the diet. Moles and warts, for example, are signs that excess protein (usually from animal sources) is being discharged. Freckles and age spots are caused by the discharge of simple sugars. Hard calluses on the hands and feet develop from the overintake of animal protein and fat. They block the flow of energy along the meridians in the hands and feet, and diminish the flow of energy to the internal organs.

To recover from skin disorders naturally, it is helpful to minimize the intake of animal food and eat primarily vegetable foods, at least until the condition improves. It is also helpful to avoid the intake of raw or uncooked food, including raw salads and fruit. Quick, lightly cooked vegetables can be eaten instead along with a balanced diet of whole grains, beans, bean products, sea vegetables, and other whole natural foods.

Sexual and Reproductive Disorders Deposits of mucus and fat in and around the reproductive organs are the primary cause of sexual dysfunction, along with gynecological and prostate disorders. A second major cause is the overconsumption of fruits, sugars, alcohol, spices, and other expansive foods that weaken vitality. If you have lines or splits at the tips of your fingers or around the nails, that is evidence of problems in the reproductive organs. If these lines are more pronounced on the right hand, then the trouble is located in the right ovary or testicle. If the left side is worse, the organs on the left side are troubled.

In Oriental medicine, buckwheat was traditionally used to restore sexual vitality. It can be eaten from time to time along with other whole grains, either in the form of whole buckwheat, or kasha, or in the form of buckwheat noodles, or soba. Root vegetables, including burdock and wild mountain potato, or *jinenjo* (a completely different species than regular potato), also strengthen sexual vitality. Hokkaido pumpkin (a form of hard winter squash) and the leafy tops of root vegetables like daikon, carrot, and turnip are also good, as are azuki and black soybeans. To reduce an overactive sexual appetite, try foods such as cooked shiitake mushrooms, tofu, and quickly cooked leafy green vegetables.

Balancing Yin and Yang

Healing is a natural, unlearned ability. This innate human capacity is a reflection of the order of the universe, most notably, the tendency that all things have to seek harmony or balance. In simple terms, health is based on the dynamic balance between yin and yang in all aspects of life.

In *Anatomy of an Illness*, Norman Cousins describes how he recovered from ankylosing spondylitis through the use of humor, positive thinking, and vitamin C. His story illustrates how the adjustment of yin and yang in body and mind can produce self-healing. Ankylosing spondylitis is an inflammation of the lower spine that results in a fusion of the vertebrae. It is caused by an accumulation of yang, or contracting energy deep within the body. Humor, positive thinking, and vitamin C stimulate the opposite, more upward or expansive energy in the body. Although they did not cure the underlying imbalance that led to disease, these measures helped Cousins temporarily neutralize or counteract the buildup of extreme yang energy and thus led a remission of his disease.

In modern terms, the condition of harmony in the human body is referred to as *homeostasis*, from the Greek *homios*, meaning "similar," and stasis, meaning "position." During the latter part of the nineteenth century, the French physiologist Claude Bernard laid the foundation for the modern understanding of homeostasis when he demonstrated that the internal environment of living things needs to remain constant in spite of changes in the external environment. He stated that, "It is a fixity of the *millieu interior* [internal environment] which is the condition of free and independent life."

Although the body's internal condition remains fairly constant, homeostasis is not a static process. A complex array of biological and energetic processes are constantly working to maintain internal stability. Far from being static, homeostasis is actually a dynamic equilibrium, in which stability is maintained in the midst of constant internal and external change. Homeostasis is more than just a mechanical process, however. It involves the interaction between mind and body, spirit and matter, and energy and physical form. All of these aspects need to be balanced for homeostasis to be complete.

Medical science now recognizes that many sicknesses are actually self-limiting, which means that the body's power of natural healing is capable of correcting the imbalance without outside interference. Up to 90 percent of patients who seek medical attention are thought to be suffering from such conditions. These disorders serve to correct imbalance and restore the body to a condition of homeostasis. They serve a beneficial purpose in that they help the body get rid of excess, and protect it from serious trouble. These natural adjustments usually run their course once the discharge has been completed. A good example is the common cold. It is only when the body's systems for neutralizing and discharging toxins break down that the situation becomes potentially life threatening. Heart disease and cancer are examples of what can happen when, over time, the body's self-cleansing mechanisms are overwhelmed. However, even chronic conditions such as these are self-limiting if they have not progressed too far and we are able to remove the physical, mental, and spiritual obstacles to self-healing.

Ultimately, healing is a process of self-realization, through which we reconnect with our inner voice, or intuition, and with the universe around us. Mobilizing intuition is the key to living in harmony with nature, maintaining our health, and recovering from illness. Intuition does not mean day-to-day consciousness or learned knowledge, which obscures deeper awareness and obstructs positive action. Intuition is the unlearned, spontaneous awareness of the order of nature, or the principle of balance according to yin and yang, and the way to live in harmony with that order. It is the foundation for a long and healthy life on this planet. In the chapters that follow, we explain how the principle of yin and yang can help unify mind, body, and spirit in our approach to health and healing.

2
Mind/Body Healing

Once I was invited to meet a well-known spiritual teacher from India. He was more than eighty and had millions of followers throughout the world. As soon as we shook hands, I saw that he had a serious heart condition. The tip of his nose was bulbous and expanded; in Oriental diagnosis, a sign of an enlarged and weakened heart. I also noticed other signs that pointed to heart trouble and saw that his condition was caused by eating too much sugar. I said to him, "Every day you are eating sugar, and that has weakened your heart. For the sake of your health, please stop eating it." He replied, "I appreciate your advice, but consciousness, not the physical body, is my main concern." I replied, "Even if consciousness is our main concern, we still need to know how to take care of the body; otherwise, it is difficult to understand what consciousness is or how it functions." His disciples were surprised at my directness. To this he answered, "I am taking care of people's consciousness and spirituality, I am not concerned with food." So finally I said, "Okay, fine, but anyway stop eating sugar."

After bowing to each other we parted. Several months later I received word that he had suffered a heart attack and died. As a result, his worldwide organization began to come apart.

This story illustrates the difficulty that people have in understanding unity between body, mind, and spirit. Many people believe that mind and body are separate, and that view influences the way they approach health and healing. On one side are those who believe that the body is the most important factor in healing and that the mind is secondary. In the extreme, the body is thought of as a machine, with replaceable parts, and health and sickness are thought to result from exclusively physical causes. According to this view, which is characteristic of modern allopathic medicine, the processes that govern healing are entirely biological or physical, and are not influenced by thoughts, emotions, or consciousness.

On the other side are people who approach life from a metaphysical, or mystical perspective. Like those with an exclusively materialistic view, people with a metaphysical view also see the mind and body as separate. They believe that the world of matter, which includes the body, is somehow less real or important than the world of mind or consciousness. Like the spiritual teacher from India, they believe spiritual progress is not influenced by physical health, and that faith, belief, or positive thinking are sufficient to overcome illness.

In reality, mind, body, and spirit are integral parts of human existence. It is impossible to separate them, and they are equally important in health and healing. The aim of holistic healing is to establish physical, mental, and spiritual harmony in the person as a whole, and not just the relief of individual symptoms. It is, therefore, educational and seeks to deepen each person's awareness of the natural order that governs health and healing. It also seeks to equip each person with the understanding and practical tools necessary to take responsibility for their own health.

The unity of mind, body, and spirit is fundamental to a holistic world view. In the sections that follow, we explore this concept in depth, beginning with the role of the mind in healing.

The Mind in Healing

Interest in the role of the mind in healing is becoming widespread today, largely as a result of the predominantly materialistic focus of modern allopathic medicine. Accounts of faith healing (such as those reported at Lourdes), research into the placebo effect, and personal accounts describing the benefits of stress reduction, humor, and positive imaging in the recovery from illness have challenged the notion of mind-body separation. That notion took root in the healing arts in the nineteenth century when allopathic doctors sought to establish scientific credibility by adopting the model of reality proposed by classical physics. In that view, based on Descartes' arbitrary separation of mind and matter, the universe is a well-oiled machine that functions according to precise mechanical laws. Having set the vast cosmic machine in motion at some unknown time in the past, God was thought to be detached from the physical universe. There was also little room for the human mind, or consciousness, in this grand mechanical scheme. Consciousness was thus placed "outside" nature, as if it existed as a part of some separate realm.

As allopathic medicine adopted this "scientific" view, healing became less of a humanistic art and more of an impersonal science. It became less spiritual and more materialistic, less comprehensive and more specialized, less natural and more artificial, and less dependent on the body's self-healing abilities and more dependent on outside intervention. Along with the new idea of the "body machine" came the notion that sickness arose from purely physical causes. Since the mind is invisible and intangible, its influence on the body—and on the process of healing—was deemed negligible. Moreover, according to this strictly materialistic framework, the mind or consciousness was thought to arise from the physical workings of the brain. Consciousness was defined in purely materialistic terms: the mind was thought to exist only because the brain existed. The human spirit was thus confined by the closed, materialistic system of nineteenth-century physics.

As this view took hold, medical science began an intensive search for the physical agents of disease. The role of the mind in determining each person's lifestyle and behavior—and thus his or her state of health—was considered less important than the role of physical agents such as bacteria or viruses. These microscopic organisms were even considered to be more important than the condition of the person as a whole, which Claude Bernard, a leading nineteenth century dissenter from this view, referred to as an individual's biological "terrain." The role of the individual in health and healing was downplayed. People were disempowered and cut off from their innate powers of healing. Health was no longer viewed as humanity's natural state, but regarded as being dependent on an individual's access to medical science and technology, thus setting in motion a cycle of codependency.

However, during the early part of the twentieth century, the theoretical model upon which this view is based began to collapse. New discoveries in the realm of physics paved the way for more comprehensive and dynamic paradigms of reality. One was the discovery that in the world of electrons, protons, and other subatomic particles, the consciousness of the observer not only influences but may also help create the phenomenon being observed. Physicist and author Fritjof Capra describes this concept in *The Tao of Physics:*

> As we penetrate into matter, nature does not show us any isolated "basic building blocks," but rather appears as a complicated web of relations between the various aspects of the whole. These relations always include the observer in an essential way. The human observer constitutes the final link in the chain of observational processes, and the properties of any atomic object can be understood only in terms of the object's interaction with the observer. This means that the classical idea of an objective description of nature is no longer valid. The Cartesian partition between the I and the world, between the observer and the observed, cannot be made when dealing with atomic matter. In atomic physics, we can never speak about nature without, at the same time, speaking about ourselves.

By reestablishing the link between consciousness and the physical universe, a link that lies at the heart of traditional cosmologies and healing systems throughout the world, this discovery revealed a major flaw in the classical world-view. Moreover, the discovery that thoughts and emotions play an important role in health and healing, a fact known by traditional healers for centuries, has revealed the limits of the model of health and disease based on the separation of mind and body. Mental relaxation, a positive view of life, a strong will to live, and good human relations have all been shown to influence the healing process. On the other hand, negative emotions, such as anxiety, depression, and fear have been found to inhibit the immune system—and our self-healing ability. Positive emotions such as love, hope, and confidence have been found to enhance immune function.

Severe emotional or psychological stress has long been associated with increased susceptibility to illness. People who have recently experienced the death of a spouse or loved one often have higher than average incidences of cancer, arthritis, infection, and other conditions. Strong feelings of grief can inhibit the immune system. In a study conducted by researchers in Australia, subjects who had recently lost a spouse were found to have diminished T-cell functioning. (T-cells are a type of lymphocyte, or white blood cell, and play an important role in the body's immune response.) In another study conducted at the Mount Sanai School of Medicine in New York, men who were married to women with advanced breast cancer were found to have a similar pattern of lymphocyte inhibition that lasted for several months following the death of their spouses. Their immune responses gradually returned to normal as their experience of bereavement eased.

The heart and circulatory system also react to stress. Studies have shown that persons with repressed anger or hostility often have higher than average blood pressures and an increased incidence of coronary artery disease. In one study of persons with blockage of the coronary arteries, those with the most severe blockage had the greatest degree of repressed anger and hostility. Persons with fewer repressed emotions had less severe disease. Those with severe arterial blockage angered easily but tended not to express their feelings.

These characteristics are common among persons with so-called "Type A" behavior. More yang Type A persons tend to be highly competitive, impatient, and constantly pressed for time. They are easy to anger, have trouble relaxing, and are prone to coronary disease. The opposite behavior pattern, labeled "Type B," is characterized by a yin, relaxed, patient, and even-tempered attitude with fewer feelings of time pressure. Persons with Type B behavior are also less prone to coronary disease.

The so-called "placebo response" is cited as an example of the power of the mind in overcoming the symptoms of disease. The Latin word *placebo* means "I will please," and usually refers to an inactive substance that is given to a patient to satisfy the need for medication. When combined with the power of positive suggestion, placebos have been found to trigger biochemical changes in the body that aid the relief of symptoms. They have been used to relieve pain, induce mental alertness, and initiate recovery from the symptoms and signs of chronic diseases. When combined with negative suggestion, they have been found to cause negative side effects that are similar to those of powerful drugs. Norman Cousins describes the implications of the placebo in his book, *Anatomy of an Illness*:

> The placebo is proof that there is no real separation between mind and body. Illness is always an interaction between both. It can begin in the mind and affect the body, or it can begin in the body and affect the mind, both of which are served by the same bloodstream. Attempts to treat most mental diseases as though they were completely free of physical causes and attempts to treat most bodily diseases as though the mind were in no way involved must be considered archaic in light of new evidence about the way the human body functions.

Biochemical Pathways

Investigators seeking to discover how the mind influences physical health have tended to focus on the biochemical pathways through which the brain influences various bodily functions. The positive expectations elicited by a placebo, for example, are thought to stimulate the cortex, which in turn activates the endocrine system, including the adrenal glands. The action of adrenal hormones in turn affects the body's organs and functions. Positive expectations may also activate the autonomic nervous system, and thus activate or inhibit various body functions. They may also stimulate the brain to secrete chemicals known as endorphins that have the effect of reducing the awareness of pain.

Thoughts, moods, and emotions also affect the brain's secretion of chemicals that carry messages between cells. These chemical messages are carried by neurohormones that travel through the bloodstream and by neurotransmitters that travel through the body-wide network of nerve cells. These chemicals are attracted to specialized receptors on the surface of body cells, and either stimulate or inhibit the activity of the cell.

The nervous and immune systems are also closely intertwined. Organs such as the spleen, bone marrow, lymph nodes, and thymus gland, where cells of the immune system develop and mature, are richly endowed with nerve endings. Moreover, immune cells contain numerous receptors for neurotransmitters, neurohormones, and neuropeptides secreted by the brain and nervous system. Thus, by stimulating the release of these chemicals, thoughts and emotions can potentially activate or inhibit the immune response.

The nervous system is not the only channel through which thoughts and emotions affect the body. Thoughts and emotions exist in the form of energy waves that travel through an invisible, body-wide network that connects each cell in the body. Until recently, modern medicine was not aware of this invisible energy system. This concept had not been encountered until investigators began to study the traditional healing systems of the East, where the body's invisible energy system was known and used for thousands of years. This system, comprised of meridians, meridian branches, and chakras, may hold the key to understanding the interaction between mind and body. After all, human consciousness is an invisible, energetic phenomenon. Trying to understand it in terms of the biochemical effects it produces is like trying to understand what someone is like by examining footprints in the sand. In order to create a truly holistic paradigm, we need to embrace and understand the traditional concept of energy. The body's energy system represents the new frontier of health and healing. It holds the key to unifying mind and body, spirit and matter, and consciousness and health.

Bioenergetic Pathways

The medical systems of India, China, Japan, and other Asian countries are based on the understanding and use of life energy. They go back thousands of years, and are derived from an ancient cosmology, or world-view, that saw all things in nature as manifestations of energy, or vibrations. Ayurveda, the ancient medicine of India, which dates back at least 5,000 years, taught that all things in the universe—from the tiniest atom to the largest galaxy—are different forms of universal consciousness or energy. In Japan and China, an invisible force, referred to as *Ki,* or *Ch'i,* was thought to permeate the universe. According to the centuries-old philosophy of Oriental medicine, Ki, or life energy, manifests in countless material and nonmaterial forms, including mind and body, heaven and earth, and spirit and matter. When it takes more inert, condensed forms, it appears as matter, and when it assumes more diffused, dynamic forms, it appears as mind, consciousness, and other nonmaterial phenomena.

The concept of life energy is basic to traditional concepts of health and healing. In Japan, for example, sickness is described as *Byo-Ki,* or "suffering Ki," meaning that illness is a manifestation of energy imbalance. Kahuna medicine, the native healing tradition of Hawaii, is founded on the same idea. The Kahuna word for good health means "abundance of energy." Poor health is conceived of either as a weakness, or lack of energy, or as tension or blockage in the flow of energy throughout the body. The word for "healing" means to restore energy and achieve a condition of harmony or fullness.

The traditional concept of energy is not incompatible with modern science. New discoveries in the realm of physics have made it possible to unite scientific understanding with this ancient view. In the view of nineteenth century physics, atoms were tiny, material points and were the final, irreducible unit of matter. However, when scientists began to subdivide and analyze atoms, they discovered that atoms are composed largely of empty space within which much smaller units known as electrons, protons, and neutrons are in constant motion. (Today, over two-hundred of these subatomic "particles" have been identified.) Moreover, when these smaller units were studied closely, it was discovered that they are not particles, but condensed packets of energy that have the characteristics of both intangible waves and tangible particles. They are material in the sense that they leave behind tracks that can be detected with the senses, and at the same time are fleeting, impermanent, and nonmaterial. Thus, according to modern physics, matter is essentially composed of energy, or nonmatter. That conclusion was reached thousands of years ago and articulated in the concept of Ki, or life energy. Again, to quote Fritjof Capra:

> All particles can be transmuted into other particles: they can be created from energy and can vanish into energy. In this world, classical concepts like "elementary particle," "material substance," or "isolated object" have lost their meaning; the whole universe appears as a dynamic web of inseparable energy patterns.

Our planet is constantly bathed in cosmic energy. From the infinite periphery of space, energy is spiraling in toward the earth in the form of solar and stellar radiation, cosmic rays, and solar and galactic wind, together with light and energy from a countless number of stars, planets, galaxies, and other celestial bodies. Because this stream of energy originates in the cosmos, we can refer to it as heaven's force. It moves from the infinite periphery of space toward the infinitesimally tiny point known as the earth, and exerts a condensing or contracting effect on the earth and everything on it. Because of its rotation, the earth also generates a tremendous amount of energy. Heaven's force pushes everything down toward the surface of the planet. Earth's force is the opposite: it spirals up from the surface of the planet and out toward infinite space. Together these forces charge the planet and everything on it. They are the primary sources of the life energy that charges all beings, and that animates every aspect of our lives, including the movements of the body, our mental and emotional responses, and our spiritual qualities.

Body, mind, and spirit are the product of these primary forces. Human life exists at the balancing point between heaven and earth. We are created by the fusion of these two huge streams of energy. In the body, they create two complementary "trees" that animate all aspects of life. One, which we can refer to as the tree of consciousness, is primarily the product of heaven's force. It is comprised of invisible energy and originates in the universe. The other, which we refer to as the tree of the body, consists of the physical, material body, including organs, tissues, and cells. The physical body is formed out of the material substance of the earth, including food, water, and air.

The Chakras

Heaven's energy spirals in toward the surface of the planet and enters the human body through the spiral, or cowlick, on top of the head. From here, energy streams downward along an invisible line running deep within the body. This primary energy channel charges the entire body and all of its functions. It extends from the top of the head to the sexual organs. Heaven's downward force enters the top of the head, flows through the body, and exits in the region of the sexual organs. Meanwhile, an invisible stream of earth's force moves along the primary channel in the opposite direction, entering in the region of the sexual organs and exiting through the hair spiral.

The Body, Chakras, and Primary Channel

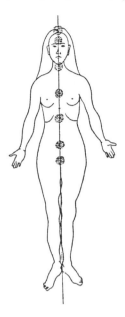

The flow of heaven's and earth's forces through the primary channel gives rise to seven highly charged energy centers, which in ancient India were named *chakras*, or spiral *wheels*. The chakras concentrate energy from the surrounding environment and distribute it throughout the body. The *crown*, or *seventh chakra* is located at the top of the head in the region of the hair spiral. Because of its position, the crown chakra is highly charged with cosmic energy and supplies this energy to the cerebral cortex, providing the basis for the images, consciousness, and sensations that arise there. Energy from this chakra radiates in a gold color.

The next energy center is located deep within the brain, in the area of the midbrain. This focal point of energy is known as the *sixth*, or *midbrain chakra*. Energy is distributed from this chakra to the millions of cells in the brain. Brain cells function as highly communicative instruments, processing vibrations in a manner similar to a television set, receiving energy from the primary channel and producing images, sensations, and consciousness. Thoughts and images take the form of invisible, vibrational holograms projected onto three-dimensional space. Energy in the midbrain chakra radiates in a silver-yellow color.

Heaven's force moves downward through the body and causes the uvula to develop at the back of the throat. It also causes a pair of glands, the adenoids, to develop in the form of spirals on either side of the uvula. Heaven's force also creates and activates the salivary glands, generating the production of a highly charged liquid, saliva. Meanwhile, earth's force—which streams upward from the lower body—creates and charges the tongue, along with a pair of glands in the throat known as the tonsils.

As it concentrates in the throat, heaven's force produces another highly charged energy center known as the *fifth*, or *throat chakra*. The concentration of energy here activates the motion of the tongue and vocal cords, producing the human voice. It also stimulates the thyroid and parathyroid glands to secrete hormones. Energy in the throat chakra radiates in a yellow color.

The *fourth*, or *heart chakra* is located in the center of the chest in the region over the heart. Here, the active rhythm of heaven's and earth's forces produces the heartbeat. Contracting of the heart is produced by heaven's force, and expansion by earth's force. The rhythmic movement of the lungs is also regulated by the energy in this chakra, and energy from this center charges the heart and circulation, blood and body fluids, and the function of breathing. Feelings and emotions, including those of love, compassion, and sympathy, are also produced here. Heart chakra energy radiates in a pink color.

The *third*, or *stomach chakra* is located in the center of the solar plexus, about two inches below the base of the sternum. It activates the movement of the stomach and digestive organs and supplies the liver, spleen, gallbladder, pancreas, and kidneys with energy. This chakra translates the images and feelings generated in the upper chakras into the movements of the lower body, and activates the secretion of hormones and digestive juices. Energy in the stomach chakra radiates in an orange color.

The *second*, or *hara chakra*, is located in the lower part of the small intestine, about two fingers below the navel, and is the central focus of energy in the lower abdomen. It is also referred to as *Ki-Kai,* or "ocean of electromagnetic energy," and *Tanden,* or the "central field" of energy. From here energy is distributed in waves, causing rhythmic expansion and contraction of the small and large intestines. Intestinal digestion, decomposition and absorption of food molecules, and movement of the intestines occur because of the energy flowing from this chakra. Hara chakra energy radiates in a red color.

Chakras and the Endocrine System

Each chakra functions as a center of consciousness. The chakras influence the body through the activity of the meridians, and through the endocrine system. Energy from the chakras either stimulates or inhibits the endocrine glands. The correspondences between the chakras and endocrine glands are presented below:

Chakra	Primary Correspondence	Secondary Correspondence
Seventh (crown) and Sixth (mid-brain)	Pituitary, pineal	Hypothalamus
Fifth (throat)	Thyroid	Parathyroid
Fourth (heart)	Thymus	Heart
Third (stomach)	Pancreas	Stomach, duodenum, adrenal, kidney
Second (hara)	Ovary	Adrenal, kidney,
First (base)	Testis	Ovary

In women, the hara chakra is located in the upper part of the uterus. It is here that implantation of the fertilized ovum takes place. The intense charge of life energy in this region stimulates development of the placenta and embryo, and after nine months activates the contractions that occur during labor. Labor begins when the charge of heaven's and earth's forces intensifies in the hara region, causing the uterus to begin rhythmic contractions.

These movements begin in the hara chakra and spread downward in the form of a wave.

The *first*, or *base chakra*, is located at the base of the spine. It charges the bladder, rectum, and reproductive organs, and activates physical and sexual vitality. Heaven's downward force exits the body through this chakra, while earth's expanding force enters the body in this region. Energy in the sexual chakra radiates in a dark red color.

The primary channel and chakras are the trunk of the tree of consciousness. The two upper chakras in the head comprise the roots of this upside-down tree. Although the central line conducts both heaven's and earth's forces, its primary energy source flows downward from the sky to the earth. On the earth, heaven's descending force is generally seven times stronger than the upward, centrifugal force generated by the rotation of the planet. Therefore, we can say that the soil that nourishes the tree of consciousness is the universe itself.

The Meridians

Like the trunk of a tree, the primary channel differentiates into branches. Each branch carries energy from the primary channel to the rest of the body. These branches are known in Oriental medicine as *meridians*. Meridians radiate outward from the primary channel in the way that the ridges of a pumpkin branch outward from the central core. Although they are usually thought of as energy "lines," each meridian is actually a spiral, with the most peripheral orbit running near the surface of the body below the skin. Each meridian-spiral coils inward so that the central orbits are located deep within the body. Here, each stream of energy differentiates into numerous smaller branches that end in billions of cells. This process occurs in seven stages, with each branch subdividing into smaller and smaller units. Like stars that cluster into constellations, cells cluster into groups that are nourished by a particular meridian. These condensed cell clusters are the internal organs. The cells of the skin, muscles, bones, brain and nervous system, and glands also differentiate from the meridians and chakras and are part of this complex energy network.

The process through which the primary channel differentiates into meridians, meridian branches, and cells is similar to the process through which the trunk of a tree differentiates into numerous branches and leaves. Just as each leaf receives nourishment from the roots of the tree, each cell is constantly supplied with energy from primary channel and chakras. Cosmic energy is constantly streaming into the body, charging each cell and animating all of its functions.

Each meridian also has numerous direct channels to the outside. These channels take the form of tiny "holes" at the surface of the body. Energy from the outside enters the body through these holes, and is absorbed and incorporated into general flow of energy along the meridian. At the same time, energy produced inside the body flows outward through these holes. Each hole is like a miniature volcano that releases energy from inside the earth. The body-wide network of energy holes comprises the system of "points" used in acupuncture, shiatsu massage, and other traditional Oriental therapies.

Although they develop through a similar process of differentiation, trees and human beings actually have an opposite structure. The roots of the tree are in the earth. Energy and nutrients from the soil stream upward through the trunk, and out through the branches to each leaf and flower. The tree's reproductive functions are carried on in the upper, most peripheral regions of the tree where flowers and seeds are produced. The roots of the human body are in the head, through which energy from the universe flows downward along the primary channel, charging the chakras, meridians, and cells. Unlike leaves that develop externally, cells appear deep inside the body. Our reproductive functions, which are similar to the fruit, flowers, and seeds of the tree, are not located in an upward position, but downward at the lower end of the primary channel. The human ovum is not fertilized externally, as seeds are, but are fertilized internally. It develops deep within the mother's body rather than separate from the mother in the outside environment.

The uppermost chakras are the first to receive the incoming flow of celestial force. Thoughts and images produced in these chakras generate energy waves that travel down the primary channel, through the chakras, and out to the meridians. Consciousness waves then disperse through the minute network of meridian branches, arriving ultimately at the cells, in a process that is similar to the transmission of nerve impulses from the brain through the finely differentiated network of peripheral nerves. The nature of these consciousness waves has a direct influence on the functioning of the cell. Each cell is influenced by the thoughts, images, and vibrations produced in the uppermost chakras.

A calm, clear, and tranquil mind allows energy to stream freely through the primary channel and chakras. Bright, happy, or positive thoughts stimulate the flow of life energy reaching the cells. Dark, negative, or depressing thoughts weaken or interfere with the smooth flow of energy along these pathways, and diminish the supply of energy reaching the cells. And as we have seen, thoughts also affect the way brain cells secrete chemical messengers, and these also affect the body's cells. The speed at which consciousness waves travel through the chakras, meridians, and meridian branches is more rapid than the speed at which impulses travel through the nervous system. As a consequence, thoughts, images, and vibrations arising in the brain influence the cells through the invisible energy network before they activate the biochemical pathways described above.

The body and mind are one. Through pathways both visible and invisible, thoughts and images exert a profound influence on our health and well-being.

Development of the Chakras

The chakra system is one of the keys to understanding the relationship between body, mind, and spirit. We are constantly receiving vibrations from our environment, both near and far. These include the full range of sensory inputs and more subtle vibrations, including those of consciousness and thinking. They travel from the periphery of the body to the brain via the nervous system. Images, thoughts, and emotions arise in response, and produce impulses that flow down the primary chakra line, charging and activating certain chakras. Depending on the type of energy that is produced, the chakras are either activated or inhibited.

The invisible energy system grows downward in a manner that is opposite to trees in the vegetable kingdom. The uppermost chakras become active early in life. They function in concert with the brain in coordinating our mechanical and sensory activities. The third, or throat chakra, becomes active soon afterward, stimulating the ability of speech and self-expression. Then, the energetic functions of the fourth, or heart chakra become active, and emotions and feelings, including those of love and tenderness, appear. Intellectual ability develops next, and this capacity is centered in the fourth, or stomach chakra in the solar plexus. As the sixth, or hara chakra becomes active, social awareness begins developing. The seventh, or sexual chakra becomes active at about the age of fourteen for girls and sixteen for boys. Sexual and reproductive abilities are the last to develop and are an extension of the capacities centered in the hara chakra. Sexuality represents the condensed essence of all social relationships.

The chakras are centers for these mental and emotional capacities. The direction in which they develop—downward from heaven to earth—is opposite to the direction in which consciousness develops. Consciousness expands upward and outward, beginning with mechanical responses to the environment, followed by sensory awareness, emotional and intellectual responses, social and philosophical concerns, and ultimately all-embracing universal consciousness. This process occurs in the form of an expanding spiral that counterbalances the contracting spiral through which human life takes form. As our consciousness develops, we are able to embrace larger and larger dimensions of time and space.

Meridians as Channels of Consciousness

The meridians begin and end in the chakras. Each one is a channel for the vibrations of consciousness produced in the chakras. The body's cells are connected to the meridians through the meridian branches, and act as thought or consciousness centers. Mind and body are one, and are unified by the body's invisible energy system. The meridians also channel energy from the environment and either activate or sedate the mental and emotional functions centered in the chakras. Below we explain the relationship between the meridians, chakras, and dimensions of consciousness. In subsequent chapters we will explore the implications of this relationship in diagnosis and treatment.

Lung Meridian/Intellect (Activating) The lung meridian begins at the stomach chakra and descends to connect with its partner organ, the large intestine. It then reverses direction, passes through the lungs, ascends to the throat, and moves out to the shoulder. From there, it runs down the inner arm to the outer corner of the thumbnail. Several inches above the wrist, a branch of the lung meridian descends directly to the index finger, where the large intestine meridian begins.

The lung meridian flows outward from the body and is charged with earth's yin energy. The intellectual capacities generated in the stomach chakra flow out along the lung meridian in the form of waves. We can say that the lung meridian is a channel for waves of intellect. The strong current of earth's expanding energy that charges the lung meridian causes the intellect to become active rather than dormant. The meridian on the right side of the body (and the right lung) is powerfully charged with earth's force, and strongly activates the intellect. The meridian on the left side of the body (and the left lung) is strongly charged with heaven's force, and has a weak activating effect on intellectuality.

Large Intestine Meridian/Social Awareness (Stabilizing) The large intestine meridian begins at the thumb-side corner of the index finger and runs up the finger, hand, and thumb side of the arm to the top of the shoulder. From here, one branch enters the body and descends to the large intestine and hara chakra. Another branch goes from the shoulder up the side of the neck to the face, crosses between the mouth and the nose, and ends at the outside corner of the nostril. At the the end of the nostril, this branch connects to the stomach meridian.

The large intestine meridian receives energy from the hara chakra, and is a channel for our social awareness. On the whole, the large intestine meridian is charged with heaven's yang force, and thus has a stabilizing, rather than an activating, effect on social development. The meridian on the right arm has a weak stabilizing effect, as does the ascending colon, while the meridian on the left arm has a more powerful stabilizing effect, as does the descending colon.

Stomach Meridian/Intellect (Stabilizing) The stomach meridian begins at the corner of the nose. One branch goes to the head, while another branch enters the body and descends to the stomach. It continues down the trunk, over the front of the thigh to the outside of the knee. Continuing downward, it runs on the outside of the lower leg over the top of the foot to the second and third toes. From the top of the foot, a branch diverts to the outside corner of the first toe. Here the spleen meridian begins.

The stomach meridian is a channel for intellectuality. It is strongly charged with heaven's force and has the effect of stabilizing, focusing, or centering intellectual activity. The stomach meridian on the right side of the body has a weak stabilizing effect, while the meridian on the left side has a strong stabilizing effect.

Spleen Meridian/Emotion, Intellect, Social Awareness (Activating) The spleen meridian begins at the outside corner of the first, or large toe, and rises along the inside of the foot above the arch around the anklebone. It ascends along the inner leg, enters the trunk and connects with the spleen. A branch of the spleen meridian goes to the three chakras in the trunk of the body, the hara chakra, the stomach chakra, and the heart chakra. A branch also ascends up the outside of the trunk and goes to the throat chakra. At the heart chakra it connects with the heart meridian.

The spleen meridian is a channel for the emotions generated in the heart chakra, the intellectuality produced in the stomach chakra, and the social awareness originating in the hara chakra. This meridian is charged with earth's ascending energy, and therefore activates these functions of consciousness. The spleen meridian on the right side of the body is highly charged with earth's rising power, and strongly activates these capacities. The meridian on the left side is less strongly charged by earth's energy and has a milder activating effect. Since it connects with the throat chakra, the spleen meridian also activates speech and other forms of vocal expression.

Heart Meridian/Emotion, Intellect (Activating) Beginning at the heart chakra, one branch of this meridian moves upward across the chest, the side of the throat and face, to the eye. Another branch goes down to the stomach chakra, and another to the armpit and down the middle of the inside of the arm to the end of the little finger on the inside. The heart meridian connects to the small intestine meridian at the end of the little finger.

The heart meridian is a channel for the emotions generated in the heart chakra and the functions of intellect originating in the stomach chakra. It is charged with earth's energy, and has an activating effect. The heart meridian on the right side strongly activates the emotions and intellect, while the meridian on the left has a weak activating effect.

Small Intestine Meridian/Emotion, Intellect (Stabilizing) The small intestine meridian begins on the outside tip of the little finger and goes back along the outside of the arm to the shoulder, where it divides into two branches. One branch goes internally down the front of the body to the small intestine, passing through the heart and stomach chakras. Another branch runs up the side of the neck to the inner corner of the eye where it connects with the bladder meridian.

The small intestine meridian acts as a channel for the emotions and intellect generated by the heart and stomach chakras. The direction of energy flow along the small intestine meridian is inward and downward, and thus it is charged primarily by heaven's yang, descending force. The small intestine meridian on the right side has a mildly inhibiting, or stabilizing effect on these mental and emotional functions, while the meridian on the left side has a strong inhibiting effect.

Bladder Meridian/ Expression, Emotion, Intellect, Social Awareness, Sexual Function (Stabilizing) The bladder meridian begins at the inner corner of the eye and runs up across the forehead, over the head and down the neck and back. The bladder meridian connects all Yu, or entrance points on the back. At the lumbar region, a branch connects to the kidney and bladder. The meridian runs down the buttocks and the back of the legs, over the outside of the Achilles tendon, around the outside of the ankle and over the foot to the outside of the little toe. From the little toe it runs to the bottom of the foot where the kidney meridian begins.

The bladder meridian does not connect directly with any of the chakras. However, the Yu points on the back are connected to all the major organs, and thus the bladder meridian is indirectly linked to the throat, heart, stomach, hara, and sexual chakras. Thus the bladder meridian serves as a channel for the functions of expression, emotion, intellect, social awareness, and sexuality produced in these chakras. The bladder meridian flows downward, and is strongly charged with heaven's force. It has the effect of stabilizing or quieting these mental and emotional functions. The bladder meridian on the right side has a weak inhibiting effect; the meridian on the left has a strong inhibiting effect. Practitioners of shiatsu often notice that hyperactive emotions can be stabilized by massaging down the bladder meridian.

Kidney Meridian/Expression, Emotion, Social Awareness, Sexual Function (Activating) The kidney meridian begins on the sole of the foot toward the front, in the indentation between the pads formed at the base of the toes. This meridian runs along the arch of the foot, circles the inner anklebone, ascends the inside of the leg, and moves through the trunk where it connects with the sexual chakra and kidney. It then continues upward to the throat, connecting with the hara, heart, and throat chakras. A branch of the kidney meridian goes to the heart chakra where it connects to the heart governor meridian.

The kidney meridian is a channel for the functions of expression, emotion, social awareness, and sexuality generated in the chakras mentioned above. The kidney meridian flows upward and is charged by earth's expanding energy. It therefore has an activating effect on these mental and emotional functions. The kidney meridian on the right side has a strong activating effect, while the meridian on the left side has a mild activating effect.

The difference between the bladder and kidney meridians, in terms of their effects on psychological and emotional functions, can be seen in the way that massaging them effects a person's thoughts and emotions. Massaging down the bladder meridian on the back stabilizes a person's energy, calms the emotions, and deactivates sexual response. A person often becomes inwardly focused and quiet after receiving massage along the bladder meridian. Massaging up the kidney meridian on the front of the body has the opposite effect. It activates the emotions and sexual response and often causes a person to become talkative.

Heart Governor Meridian/Emotion, Intellect, Social Awareness (Activating) The heart governor meridian begins in the pericardium and runs across the chest and down the inside of the arm, over the center of the palm to the tip of the middle finger. A branch extends from the center of the palm to the fourth or ring finger where the triple heater meridian begins. The heart governor meridian is connected to three of the bodily chakras: the heart, stomach, and hara, and thus serves as a channel for the emotions, intellect, and social awareness generated in these chakras. The heart governor meridian is charged by earth's expanding energy and has an activating effect on these functions. The meridian on the right side has a strong activating effect; the meridian on the left side has a mild activating effect.

Triple Heater Meridian/Emotion, Intellect, Social Awareness (Stabilizing) The triple heater meridian begins at the outside of the ring finger and runs up the outside of the arm to the shoulder. One branch continues upward over the side of the head. Another branch goes to the trunk and connects the three chakras collectively known as the triple heater—the heart, stomach, and hara chakras. The branch of the triple heater meridian that goes to the face connects with the gallbladder meridian at the end of the eyebrow.

The triple heater meridian serves as a channel for the emotional, intellectual, and social capacities generated in the heart, stomach, and hara chakras. The triple heater meridian is charged by heaven's descending energy, and has a stabilizing effect on these functions. The meridian on right side has a weak stabilizing effect; the meridian on the left side has a strong stabilizing effect.

Gallbladder Meridian/Intellect, Sexual Function (Stabilizing) One branch of the gallbladder meridian starts at the face and passes downward through the neck and chest to the gallbladder. It connects with the main branch at the hip. The main branch begins at the outside of the eyebrow and rises across the side of the head where it spirals or zigzags several times before going down the side of the neck to the top of the shoulders. It runs down the side of the trunk to the hip. From here it goes down the outside of the leg, crossing above the anklebone, and running to the fourth toe. A branch goes to the inside of the large toe where the liver meridian begins.

The gallbladder meridian does not connect directly with the chakras. In the rib cage, it indirectly connects with the stomach chakra, and in the lower abdomen, to the sexual chakra. It thus serves as a channel for the functions of intellect and sexuality produced in these chakras. The gallbladder meridian is charged strongly with heaven's force, and thus has a stabilizing effect on these functions. The meridian on the right side of the body has a mild stabilizing effect on these functions; the meridian on the left side has a strong stabilizing effect.

Liver Meridian/Intellect, Social Awareness, Sexual Function (Activating) The liver meridian begins at the inside corner of the large toe and travels up the inside of the leg, enters the trunk, and moves up to the liver. This meridian continues up the trunk to the eyes, and on to the top of the head. From here, a branch goes to the stomach chakra where it connects to the first meridian, the lung meridian.

In its course through the abdomen, the liver meridian gives

rise to a branch that connects with the sexual chakra. It also connects indirectly with the hara chakra, and branches into the stomach chakra. The liver meridian therefore serves as a channel for the functions of intellect, social awareness, and sexuality produced in these chakras. The liver meridian is strongly charged with earth's force, and has an activating effect on these functions. The meridian on the right side has a strong activating effect; the meridian on the left side has a milder activating effect.

Governing Vessel/Physical, Mental, and Spiritual Functions (Activating and Strengthening) The governing vessel begins at the coccyx and flows upward on the surface of the back, along the spinal cord, over the head and down the face to the mouth. Entering the mouth, the governing vessel descends internally to the genital area, and exits at the perineum, where the cycle begins again. The governing vessel activates and strengthens our physical, mental, and spiritual abilities, together with our power to maintain the functions of life in well-coordinated harmony.

Conception Vessel/Physical, Mental, and Spiritual Functions (Activating) The conception vessel, along with its partner, the governing vessel, constitute the body's original meridian. Together they form the primary channel, and represent the principal flow of heaven's and earth's forces within the body. Working together, they have a comprehensive influence on all physical, psychological, and spiritual functions. It is from the conception and governing vessels that the other meridians differentiate.

The conception vessel begins at the perineum, the area between the anus and genitals, and streams upward on the front surface of the body. It moves along the center of the trunk to the mouth. Entering the mouth, the conception vessel moves down the center of the body, deep inside. It exits in the area of the coccyx, the small triangular bone at the base of the spine, where it connects with the governing vessel. The conception vessel activates our spiritual, mental, and physical functions. When energy is flowing smoothly through the conception vessel, a person feels uplifted, activated, and eager to accomplish something.

The Tree of the Body

The tree of the body is rooted in the earth and complements the invisible tree of consciousness. Consciousness is primarily a product of heaven's force, while the body is assembled from material substance of the earth.

On earth, the vegetable kingdom combines with elements, including air, water, and minerals, to provide the physical substance of the body. If we compare the body to the clay on a potter's wheel, heaven's energy creates the motion of the wheel and acts like invisible hands that shape the clay. Heaven's force charges the entire body; it is the primary source of the life energy that streams into every cell. The body itself is composed of the material substance of the earth and is like the clay being shaped by the potter's fingers.

Like the invisible energy system, the body is formed in a way that is opposite to trees and other forms of plant life. A tree absorbs nutrients from the soil through external roots. The roots of the body are deep inside in the small intestine. It is here that nutrients are absorbed into the bloodstream and distributed to the body's cells. The branched structure of the circulatory system resembles the branched structure of a tree. At the most peripheral part, nutrients diffuse through minute capillaries into the cells. Cells are like the leaves of a tree. However, leaves develop externally and are open and expanded, while cells develop internally and are closed and compact.

Each cell is nourished by two complementary streams: one, the invisible stream of energy that enters the cell via meridian branches, and the other, the physical stream of nourishment entering the cell from the bloodstream. These streams move in opposite directions; one spirals from the diffuse world of energy toward the condensed world of matter, and the other spirals from the condensed world of matter toward the world of energy. Everyone more or less receives the same general influence from the universe, although everyone occupies a unique position in time and space and channels heaven's energy from a slightly different perspective. Individual differences are primarily a result of differences in the foods that people select. Food creates the unique composition of each cell. The unlimited variation in food choices creates the endless variety of physical constitutions and conditions found among people.

When a tree grows in healthy soil, it receives balanced nourishment and is able to thrive. But if the soil is deficient in minerals or contaminated with chemical toxins, the tree becomes unhealthy and its leaves eventually wither and die. A naturally balanced diet is like healthy soil. It provides the body with proper nourishment, thus ensuring sound blood and healthy functioning of each cell. If food becomes unbalanced, the blood begins to deteriorate, and cells become unhealthy. The leaves of the tree depend on nutrients absorbed through the roots. Cells, including those of the brain and nervous system, depend on the nutrients passing through the small intestine. Body and mind are both nourished by the same bloodstream. By influencing the blood and cells, daily foods profoundly influence our physical health, together with our consciousness and emotions.

Consciousness and Brain Function

The development of consciousness parallels activation of a wider region of the brain. The brain has three main divisions: the cerebrum, which governs our thinking and judgment; the cerebellum, which is yang (being toward the rear of the head and having a compact structure), which governs our activity; and the midbrain, which regulates the two and provides a smooth interchange between them. The midbrain is the generator of our intelligence and intuition. Nerve impulses that are transmitted to the brain pass through the midbrain, enter the cerebrum, where they are evaluated, and through the cerebellum, where they are translated into appropriate action. From here, they activate the proper nerves so that we can respond in the manner that is best for our survival and happiness. If the functioning of these organs is rough, we are not able to judge and act the way we should.

Poor eating disturbs the brain centers. For example, if we take too much sugar, fruit, coffee, alcohol, or other strongly yin foods or drinks, they are attracted to the yang cerebellum, which will enlarge and begin to function poorly. As a result, we become less active, since the cerebellum governs our ability to change thinking into action.

The brains of animals are similar to ours, but less developed. Impulses cannot pass deeply into the cerebrum. They are much more honest than we are, and are rarely sick. As human beings, we have the ability to develop ourselves endlessly, but with that goes the privilege of making ourselves sick and unhappy.

The deeper into the cerebrum the impulses pass, the higher the consciousness that is being used. If an immediate, mechanical response is sufficient, the impulse will bypass the cerebrum altogether, such as when we jerk our hand away from something hot. From here, the brain develops upward and forward, and these regions are where the higher consciousness centers are located. The first layer is mainly concerned with the senses. Our first reaction, then, is usually to please our sensory understanding. Next come the emotions, which comprise our sentimental consciousness. If we think more deeply (notice how our language expresses what is actually a physical reality), we judge and act by our intellectual consciousness. Here we pass beyond sensory gratification and emotional fulfillment alone, and begin to search for understanding that can lead to lasting happiness.

As we develop further; our social awareness begins to emerge, which is beyond intellectuality, with a much deeper understanding of life's purpose. People with developed social awareness can solve the problems of humanity, which intellectuals and inventors cannot. Beyond this, we begin to penetrate into the regions of ideological or philosophical understanding, and our consciousness embraces almost everything. At this stage we are concerned with justice and injustice, righteousness and unrighteousness, or with some type of discipline or practice. To the extent that we remain at this level, we are not yet truly free. When our highest capacities begin to unfold, we pass beyond the limited, relative world of duality and attain all-embracing, universal consciousness. In our daily lives, these forms of consciousness operate as follows:

1. An immediate, momentary, and simultaneous response, a mechanical reaction that does not call the cerebrum into play.
2. Sensory discrimination and response, such as eating only for the purpose of satisfying hunger (using a small part of the cerebrum).
3. Sentimental feeling and response, such as most romantic imagination and behavior (using a little larger area of the cerebrum).
4. Intellectual discrimination and response, such as the formation of abstract theories, systems, and related forms of reasoning (using further extended areas of the cerebrum).
5. Wider and more practical thinking, or social understanding, including the interrelationships between humanity and the natural world (using higher and wider territories of the cerebrum).
6. Ideological or philosophical imagination, which forms the thoughts, principles, ideas, and beliefs that see causes, effects, and their processing mechanisms (using more control and peripheral areas of the brain).
7. Universal, spiritual, and all-embracing free consciousness (using all parts of the brain in coordinated harmony).

Life is a continual process of self-discovery in which our consciousness develops endlessly. When we live in harmony with this process, we go in the same direction as the movement of the universe, and embrace larger and larger circles of life. Health and well-being are the natural result of living in harmony with this universal current. Ultimately, the aim of holistic healing is to help everyone reestablish harmony with the movement of life and develop the highest consciousness.

Evolution of Consciousness

The body is divided into two complementary regions: the expanded body and the compact head. The body deals primarily with the physical world, and the head deals with consciousness. The complementary/antagonistic nature of these two functions can be seen in their respective centers—the brain, the yang center of consciousness, is in complementary opposition to the intestines, which are the more yin center of physicalness.

Development in both areas always proceeds together, so that as biological evolution occurred, so did the evolution of consciousness. Consciousness and physical development maintain a constant balance, and this is a reflection of the balance between yin and yang found throughout nature. If one area loses balance, we have either physical or mental illness.

The first four levels of the spiral of materialization (described in Chapter 1)—the human and animal world; the world of plants; the world of elements; and the world of preatomic particles—comprise only a small part of the larger world of vibrations and energy. We need only the few sense organs and the mouth to take in the material of the physical world. But to take in the millions of vibrations of the non-physical world, we need more receptors. The vertebrae of the spine serve this purpose, as does the skin. Numerous energy receptors that feed into the meridians and chakras are located in the skin. The midbrain developed through centripetal force, and is stronger than the centrifugal, yin spiral centered in the hara, or small intestine chakra. Thus our nervous center is fine and condensed, a compact yang center, which can be seen in the minute bundles of nerve fibers it contains.

We use the complementary structures of the nervous and physical systems to balance the visible and invisible worlds. Space is yin, and the yang nervous system is more involved in dealing with space. Time is yang, and the physical body deals primarily with it. In the world of consciousness, there is little concept of time, it barely exists in our image. The concept of time is virtually erased in the consciousness system. The function of space, on the other hand, is virtually erased in the physical system.

If we view the evolutionary development of consciousness we can understand this process clearly. A spark occurs in the primordial gaseous cloud of elements that comprise the earth about 3.2 billion years ago. A great electromagnetic charge is released and the elements fuse into organic compounds. The first self-replicating strands of DNA developed in this primordial environment. DNA is composed of two coiled strands linked by nucleotide bases. One strand is yang and is charged by heaven's force, and the other is yin and charged by earth's force.

Through the activity of DNA, the forces of heaven and earth directed the aggregation of organic compounds into cells. At that time, consciousness was nothing but the consciousness of the total universe working mechanically. Elements combined according to their yin and yang natures, based on the attraction of opposites and repulsion of likes. The combination of hydrogen, which is yang, with oxygen, which is yin, gave rise to water. The earth at that time was covered with water, and in that aquatic environment, the combination of yin oxygen with carbon and hydrogen (both of which are yang) gave rise to the first molecules of carbohydrate, and in turn to primitive algae and water moss. The combination of carbon and hydrogen (both yang) with oxygen and nitrogen (both yin) gave rise to the first amino acids and proteins, leading to the development of invertebrates composed largely of water and protein. Gradually, as minerals began to appear on the earth, the water covering the planet's surface became salty, and in this environment, seaweeds developed, along with vertebrates composed of water, protein, and minerals. That was the age of fish.

As the earth continued changing, minerals gathered toward the center of the planet, water appeared at the periphery, and air expanded outward. About 400 million years ago, intense geological changes, including volcanic activity, formed islands, and large masses of dry land eventually appeared. Land provided an environment for the development of primitive land mosses and amphibians. The first amphibians were small, but with an expansive time in the solar system, large amphibians and eventually reptiles appeared, leading to the age of dinosaurs and huge, ancient plants. The atmosphere was extremely humid and global temperatures were higher than they are today. Then, about 100 million years ago, the atmosphere started to cool and the giant reptiles and lush vegetation covering the earth could no longer survive. The age of mammals began, accompanied by the rise of contracted, modern species of plants. Then, the development of tree fruits led to the appearance of monkeys and apes, and with the development of cereal grains, our first human ancestors appeared on earth.

If we trace the faculties apparent in each period, we see that sensory capacities arose in the age of fish, amphibians, and reptiles, emotional responses in the age of mammals, and intellectual abilities in the age of apes and man. The force that creates mechanical understanding is totally external. A mechanical response is spontaneous and immediate, and does not involve internal processing of stimulation received from the environment. Sensory perceptions involve both external stimulation and internal responses. As biological life became more complex, the ability to process external stimulation increased, and this led to the development of the higher levels of consciousness.

During the course of evolution, the atmosphere became colder and the earth contracted in response. The atmosphere gradually became clearer. Cold produces contraction, and life has become progressively more complex and highly organized, or yang. The human nervous system is the most yang of all: it is capable of receiving and processing the widest possible range of vibrations, both near and far. Our nervous system evolved in the form of an inwardly contracting spiral with seven complete orbits, and that structure made it possible for consciousness to progress beyond the stages that came before and toward the intellectual, social, and spiritual levels unique to human beings.

As the atmosphere gradually cleared, celestial influences became stronger. The widening range of celestial influences provided the impetus for life to become increasingly complex. With the appearance of more intense celestial radiation, increasingly complex forms of food appeared, man stood erect, and consciousness evolved and changed greatly. These developments provided the background for the appearance of human consciousness in all of its dimensions. We can see how celestial energies influence consciousness from the following example.

The earth's rotation creates two twelve-hour cycles with midnight and noon at the two complementary opposite poles. When the earth faces the sun, we feel more positive, outgoing, and energetic. During the night, we experience the negative and retreating aspects of consciousness. These two attributes reflect the differences in vibration received by the earth from the sun during the day and from the Milky Way at night. A person who is active during the day is more social and positive. A person active during the evening is inclined more toward artistic or mental activities.

You can try an experiment for yourself in order to get a better idea of how consciousness appears in each succeeding stage of evolution. Alternately assume the face down position of the reptile, an all-fours position of the mammal, a half-standing position of the ape, and finally, the erect posture of a human being. In each position, try to bring into mind memories of the past; hopes, wishes, or dreams of the future, and self-reflection in the present. Also, try to utter sounds in each position. Note your reactions in each position and mental posture.

Left-Right Balance

The midbrain is the central point of the brain, to which all vibrations are continually assembled and then dispatched in the form of nerve impulses. The balance between left and right sides of the brain is parallel to the surface of the earth. This balance is relative in nature, and deals with space. The brain contains major ridges or indentations that are formed by contraction. These ridges represent the periods of extreme cold in the history of humanity, and the development of the nervous system and consciousness in response to a cold climate. The fact that these ridges do not run evenly and parallel can be attributed to periodic axis shifts of the earth. Thus we see how coldness and the axis shifts caused the human brain to develop. Of course, changes in food played an important role in this development.

The left and right hemispheres of the brain balance the forces of heaven and earth as they manifest at the surface of the planet. The right hemisphere, and the right side of the body as a whole, receives a stronger charge of earth's yin, or expansive energy. The left side receives a stronger charge of heaven's descending force. As a result, the right hemisphere generates aesthetic, intuitive, and other more yin forms of thought and image. The left hemisphere is where yang rational or analytical thinking is produced.

The inner regions of the brain (corresponding to the center of the head) are yang, and are where our intellectual and motion centers are found. The yin, peripheral regions are where emotions arise. There is no clear borderline, but these are rather general areas. Movement toward the center produces yang, intellectual thinking, while movement toward the periphery produces yin, emotional responses. We move between these poles by making ourselves more yin or yang in our condition. For example, people who eat plenty of fruit (which is yin) tend to be more emotional and talk a great deal. Yang people tend to be quieter and involved more in activity and accomplishment.

Solving Emotional Problems

There are two fundamental solutions to emotional problems. You can either make yourself yin, and solve the problem with words, or make yourself yang and solve the problem through action. We call this kind of solution through open or frank expression honesty. Honesty can be described as expressing publicly exactly the same feelings and consciousness you feel by yourself, or within yourself. Today, many people are unable to express their true feelings, because of fear that causes them to hide their inner selves. Hiding one's true feelings requires energy and produces tension in body and mind. Thus, defensiveness arises to protect position, reputation, or pride. However, we need to ask ourselves, what is this self or "I" that we seek to protect? From birth, we are continually changing, so that in reality there is no permanent "I" to protect. We are like a waterfall continually changing and never the same from moment to moment. However, we often find ourselves hanging on to what we feel is a permanent "I." That is due primarily to physical rigidity and stagnation in our body and brain. Fear and rigidity are the product of our own sickness and illusion, and arise from a narrow view of reality.

In order to realize that we have nothing to protect and nothing to be ashamed of, we need to physically relax. Massaging the neck and shoulders is especially helpful in this regard, as is massaging downward along the spine (massaging upward causes energy to gather toward the brain and increases mental tension). The meditation, visualization, and chanting practices described later in this chapter are also helpful in relaxing tension and dissolving stagnation. As you begin feeling more relaxed, try to be open with your friends and family members. Express your feelings honestly, and talk about something you have been hiding for a long time. If you eat well and practice these simple techniques, it will become much easier to overcome guilt and fear and to communicate your innermost feelings.

Front-Back Balance

The left-right balance deals mainly with the first two levels of consciousness (mechanical and sensory). Our sense organs are all paired, and make balance between left and right. Our initial development takes place through our sensory awareness and encompasses the first two levels of understanding. Front and back development occurs next, encompassing the third (emotional) and fourth (intellectual) levels.

The back part of the brain is contracted or yang, and the

front is yin or expanded. The front-back balance deals more with time than with space. The back part of the brain is where memories of the past arise, while the front is where our vision of the future is created. Short-range planning is yang, while long-range dreams are yin. If you eat more yang foods, your short-range plans are concrete, while your future dream is less clear. If you eat more yin foods, short-range plans are less concrete, while your future dream becomes clear. Also, if you are yang, memory becomes crystal clear, while a yin condition tends to blur your memories. The first two levels of consciousness, mechanical and sensory, are served by animal foods. Our development in these areas occurs in the mother's womb where we are nourished by her bloodstream, and after birth when we take mother's milk. The sentimental and intellectual levels are served by vegetable foods. After we are no longer being fed by our mothers, we begin to develop our functions on these third and fourth levels. As we begin to eat vegetable foods, we begin to encompass the dimension of past and future, including emotional and intellectual understanding.

Four Lines of Front-Back Balance

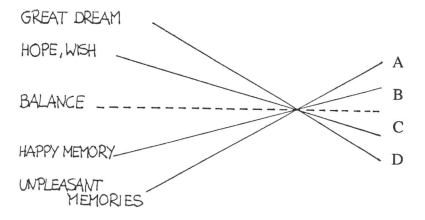

Memory and futuristic thinking are largely a function of posture, especially the angle and position of the head. When we recall the past, we tend to look downward, and when we envision the future, we raise our heads to allow the future thinking part of the brain to be up and receive vibrations. If we tilt our heads in the various up and down positions indicated in the diagram, we can see what kind of images are produced. Looking downward at a steep angle (A) brings darker or unpleasant memories, while looking slightly downward (B) brings happier, brighter memories. If we envision the future, looking slightly upward (C) brings more immediate hopes and wishes, while look upward at a steep angle (D) is conducive to great lifetime dreams.

If we eat a diet based on extreme yang animal foods, the front-back balance does not develop fully. Unpleasant memories tend to linger in our consciousness and influence our thinking and behavior. To remedy this, we need to base our diet around foods of vegetable origin that are yin in comparison to animal products. A plant-based diet helps us to develop positive images of the future. Also, as the internal organs begin to heal, posture improves so that it is difficult to keep your head lowered in the position conducive to unpleasant memories. If you have dark memories, a naturally balanced diet can help you to dispel them. Communication also furthers the healing process. If you are able to recall your most unpleasant memories and communicate them to close friends, you will be better able to discharge and let go of them.

We can now see how yang types of people are more traditional and practical and rooted to their past. Yin people, on the other hand, tend to be concerned with the future. The following practice can help you develop a positive image of the future. Sit quietly and relax. Breathe deeply and look upward at a steep angle (D in the diagram). Either close your eyes or gaze into the sky in the distance and imagine your largest dream of the future. Try to cultivate an image of health and peace, not only for yourself, but for all of humanity, and then share your visions and dreams with your friends.

Balancing Heaven and Earth

The next line of balance is not horizontal but vertical. It encompasses the social and philosophical levels of consciousness, and elevates our awareness beyond superficial or immediate concerns. This line of balance traverses the infinitesimal from the earth to the infinite of the heavens. In order to develop this level of consciousness, we eat neither animal nor vegetable food exclusively, but we eat macrobiotically, selecting the appropriate balance from among all foods for each particular person, climate, and geography. The key to this level of consciousness is the quality of our food.

The vertical line of balance actually runs from the center of the Milky Way galaxy to the other end in infinite space. It can also be called in man the primary channel, traveling from the spiral on top of the head down through our bodies. And as we saw above, we can locate seven highly charged energy centers along this channel.

Our consciousness develops along these three lines of balance: left and right, front and back, and up and down. The two horizontal balance lines represent only the relative world. The balance needed to make our thinking universal is the vertical one. To an intellectual person, this balance is called *universal law* or *justice*. To an emotional person, it is called *universal love*. We choose one of these, and adapt our expression and action to this. The vertical balance represents the consciousness of humanity. Further, in terms of human consciousness, acting on the higher vertical levels of balance is called *intuition*, while acting on the lower levels of consciousness is called *instinct*.

The vertical line gives us the objective perspective of true self-evaluation. We can see ourselves as we really are. Both our great and incredible possibilities and qualities, and our smallness, foolishness, and shortness of life become apparent. Unless we fully develop both the horizontal lines of balance, together with the vertical line of balance, we cannot experience the development of consciousness in its fullest dimensions.

The macrobiotic way of eating is to establish balance in both the horizontal and vertical lines, so we can control our kinds of thoughts, memories, and dreams by the types of food we eat. Meditation arises from the attempt to self-evaluate or to balance the vertical channel between heaven and earth. Meditation includes such practices as chanting, breathing and focusing vision, and posture. Chanting is the condensed form of modern psychology, and for thousands of years has been used to achieve balance. Chanting stabilizes the left-right balance; breathing and focusing vision achieves the front-back balance. The vertical balance is achieved by the up and down posture of meditation, which gives us empty mind or nothingness. In this state of emptiness, the forces of heaven and earth and the infinite universe fully charge our consciousness and intuition. Together with balanced eating, these practices help develop your consciousness, clear your primary energy channel, and allow your intuition to function freely without interference.

Intuition and Health

Each of us has the innate capacity to establish harmony with the movement of life, and to achieve health and happiness. This innate capacity is sometimes referred to as our intuition, and it functions on a much deeper level than day to day or surface consciousness, which is based mostly on the sensory and emotional levels. This deeper awareness includes the dreams, understanding, and images that we all have as human beings, and tends to surface during times of crisis. It provides the basis for self-reflection and change, and functions as an internal compass that keeps us aligned with nature.

This internal compass, or intuition, alerts us to potentially life-threatening habits or patterns of behavior, and includes the will to live and instinct for survival. It also motivates us to change these habits. Its source is the infinite universe itself, beyond the duality of the relative world. It functions as the universal subconsciousness within which the six levels of relative consciousness appear and disappear like waves in the ocean. Beyond differences in nationality, race, religion, or social standing, we all have this basic awareness.

Changing the cause of illness requires that we change the underlying factors that produce it. Actually, if our intuition is functioning properly, we are able to avoid the extremes that lead to illness. This intuitive capacity is native to everyone, but usually becomes dulled through improper eating and conceptual thinking. Recovering intuition is the basis for self-healing, and for maintaining harmony in body, mind, and spirit.

For example, a diet high in animal food, which is high in cholesterol and saturated fat, is the direct cause of heart disease and many forms of cancer. However, if we wish to understand the origin of these conditions on a deeper level, we need to ask why someone eats this way. Even if the underlying energy imbalance is corrected through changes in diet and lifestyle, or through such temporary measures as medication or surgery, the problem will return or reappear in another form unless the origin is changed. Changing the origin of illness requires that we change our view of life to reflect greater harmony with the universe. It also requires that we see ourselves as the cause of our problems and take responsibility for our health. Sickness arises when our intuitive awareness of the order of the universe becomes clouded. Our intuition keeps us on course with the movement of nature. When it functions properly, we intuitively know what to eat and how to live to maintain health. Sickness is actually an opportunity to reflect on our life as a whole and bring it into closer alignment with nature. In order for fundamental healing to occur, we need to change our view of life and free ourselves from the concepts and illusions that block our intuition. Understanding that we are the primary cause of our difficulties is the first step in realizing that we have the power to change our situation for the better.

The Survival Response

The twin branches of the autonomic nervous system—the sympathetic and parasympathetic nervous systems—control the body's automatic functions. The size of the pupil, for example, is automatically regulated by the amount of light. The heart is automatically beating. When food enters the stomach, digestive movements begin automatically. This system is also of great importance to overall health and the ability to resist or overcome disease.

The nerves of the parasympathetic nervous system are yang, and those of the sympathetic nervous system are yin. They affect the organs in a complementary and antagonistic way. In the stomach, the body portion is yin or expanded, while the sphincter is contracted or yang. When the parasympathetic nerves act on the stomach, the body will contract and the sphincter expand. When the sympathetic nerves act, the body of the stomach expands and the sphincter contracts. The pupil is yang or contracted. When parasympathetic nerves act on it, it will open; when sympathetic nerves act, it closes. Our body is governed by simple expansive and contractive, or yin and yang processes such as these.

Both systems are affected by what we eat and drink, and by the environment. They are influenced by what we hear, see, by colors, brightness, darkness, taste, and emotion. These systems are always reacting. As we know from experience, emotions can either stop or activate digestion. When you lose your love, for example, you cannot eat. A broken heart means that your condition has become yin because of separation. You are depressed. You do not have active, positive feelings. Instead they are negative or down. The parasympathetic nervous system is especially responsive to yin conditions such as these. When the parasympathetic nervous system acts, the stomach contracts. You lose your appetite and do not want to eat.

If you are continuously taking strong yin—such as alcohol, sugar, or medications—or strong yang—such as meat and refined salt—this mechanism will not work. Coordination is out of order. Then rigidity and one-sidedness arise. When a person uses drugs, which are extremely yin, the pupil becomes enlarged. Drugs especially weaken the parasympathetic nervous system. If someone has taken medication for a long time, their autonomic nervous system is in trouble. Reactions slow down. Orderliness disappears. People feel no need for order or cleanliness when their autonomic nervous system is sick, out of order, and no longer alert.

Being able to respond quickly—physically and emotionally—means that the autonomic nervous system is sound. If it is dull, we cannot respond, feel, and appreciate. That is sickness, and it is common now. Many people are unable to respond instinctively to changes in the environment. The autonomic nervous system is the motor of mechanical consciousness, the first level of consciousness. The mechanical level is the most important of the seven levels of consciousness. It is the foundation of life, and if it becomes dull, all the other levels will be affected. In order to make the autonomic nervous system strong, able to react quickly, eating well is especially important, as is thorough chewing. Physical and mental activity strengthen the autonomic response, as do coldness and difficulties. If you are in a situation where you have to survive, your instincts automatically become sharper. The autonomic nervous system is weakened by drugs and medications, inactivity, extreme foods, too much central heating, and a lack of contact with nature. When this system becomes dull, you cannot live in this universe, which is constantly changing. You cannot cope with the challenge of living in nature.

Weak reactivity in the autonomic nervous system is widespread in the modern world. When this system becomes dull, a person can eat extreme foods or ingest poison and have no reaction. If someone with a healthy autonomic nervous system ingests poison, he will immediately vomit or have diarrhea. His discharging powers are strong. If your autonomic responses are sound and you eat a hamburger, several hours later you will vomit or have diarrhea, or feel ill and want to eliminate it. If someone with a strong autonomic nervous system takes medication or refined sugar, he may even vomit before it enters the stomach. These reactions are normal when you are in good health. The autonomic response is one of the body's most important means of self-protection, as we can see in the following story.

About thirty years ago, a big scandal occurred in Japan. An association of businesswomen from all over Japan held a meeting at the home of their president. Cocktails were served, and some of the women drank it, others did not. Several minutes later, several of the women who had had a cocktail started to feel pain, and collapsed one by one. Ambulances were called, and several women died on the way to the hospital. Others died at the hospital, and several managed to survive after having their stomach pumped. Then the police started to check the list of the women who had attended the meeting. One woman was still unaccounted for. The police tried calling home, but there was no answer. Investigators later discovered that the president's husband had wanted to murder his wife and had put poison in the cocktail.

The police located the missing woman on the following day. They asked her where she had been the day before. She replied that she had attended the dinner party and had drunk the cocktail, after which she immediately felt nauseous. She excused herself and went to look for the bathroom. The house was a large mansion and the bathroom was some distance from the dining room. After vomiting for several minutes, she remained in the bathroom until she felt better. When she returned to the dining room, it was empty. The room was a mess but there were no people there. So she put on her coat and left. Since it was still early, she decided to go shopping. After that she went to the cinema. She had been eating macrobiotically for a number of years and was healthy and sensitive. Her body had rejected the poison. She had survived because her autonomic reactions were good.

Faith Healing and Miracle Cures

The reactions of the autonomic nervous system can help us understand the mechanism of faith healing, the placebo response, and so-called miracle cures, such as those at Lourdes, the grotto in France that is considered by many to be a holy place. About two million people visit Lourdes every year. Approximately thirty thousand of these are sick and seeking relief from their illness. For many, going to Lourdes is their last hope. Naturally, the pilgrimage to Lourdes involves a tremendous amount of mental preparation, along with the investment of time and energy.

Many people suffer from yin disorders that develop because of the overintake of extremes such as sugar, fruit, soft drinks, chocolate, spices, and chemically treated foods, or from the repeated use of drugs or medications. These yin extremes are especially harmful to the yang parasympathetic nervous system. As this system becomes weaker due to these extremes, it loses sensitivity, and this creates imbalance in the autonomic nervous system as a whole. Imbalance in the autonomic nervous system interferes with the functions of the organs and glands, and can trigger a variety of symptoms. A small number of people with this condition experience spontaneous remission at Lourdes. The rigors involved in making the trip, plus their strong confidence in the possibility of finding a cure, make the parasympathetic nervous system more yang. Some of these patients participate in the religious ceremonies at Lourdes, including plunging into a cold spring. Being in cold water produces a rapid contraction of the parasympathetic nervous system, contributing to the overall yangizing effect of the experience. Once the autonomic nervous system returns to a normal balance, the person's symptoms may quickly disappear. According to some investigators, the longer and more difficult the trip, the better the chances are of this type of remission occurring. Some researchers point out that there have been no documented cures of people who live in or near Lourdes.

Another type of spontaneous recovery occurs when a person

is experiencing more yang symptoms resulting from the overconsumption of eggs, chicken, cheese, meat, fish, and other foods from animal sources. These foods cause the body to become tense and rigid, and block the flow of energy through the chakras and meridians. A person with this condition keeps his emotions and feelings inside and cannot express himself freely. When someone is tight and tense, they feel better when they experience some type of emotional release such as crying. An overly yang condition disturbs the normal functioning of the yin sympathetic nervous system, thus producing a variety of symptoms. For many, the religious ceremonies and pageantry at Lourdes generate a great deal of emotional intensity. In this environment, a person can easily let go of egocentric attachments and submit to the will of God or the universe. For some people, the emotional release triggered by these experiences causes the sympathetic nervous system to suddenly relax, thus producing remission.

These processes underlie many instances of faith healing, along with the placebo response. The confidence generated by the placebo or by the authority of the faith healer can sometimes focus the patient's energy enough to make an overly yin parasympathetic nervous system become more yang. This effect is heightened by the person's sense that he is taking action to change his condition. In the opposite type of response, a person submits his ego to the healer or the promise inherent in the placebo, thus relaxing an overly tight sympathetic nervous system.

Although these responses can trigger a remission of symptoms in certain cases, in others they do not. For many people, measures such going to Lourdes, visiting a faith healer, or taking a placebo are not sufficient to correct imbalance in the autonomic nervous system. Unless the person reflects and changes his diet and way of life, these measures by themselves do not change the underlying cause of illness. As a result, underlying imbalance may resurface at some future time in another form. And, they do not necessarily foster a sense of self-responsibility for one's health. Unless the patient deeply reflects and changes, he may become dependent on outside intervention, rather than on his own inner resources, as the source of health and healing.

Creating a Positive Image

Thoughts and emotions can influence the healing process either negatively or positively. In order for consciousness to work positively, we need to clear the mind of negative thoughts and images, and replace them with positive ones. Positive images mobilize the will to live and liberate healing energy. Liberated energy stimulates the immune response and allows healing to occur naturally. This process is enhanced when a person understands the underlying dietary and lifestyle causes of his illness, and knows that it is possible to change these causes. The person is thus empowered by the possibility of taking positive action to change his condition.

Conversely, lack of awareness of the fundamental cause of illness leads to a sense of hopelessness and despair, especially when a person receives a negative prognosis. The fear, anxiety, and depression that result from a negative prognosis produce a sense of powerlessness that can actually diminish the possibility of recovery. Hopelessness and despair inhibit the functioning of the immune system and cause life energy to stagnate. They also diminish the will to live. Norman Cousins describes this effect in the book *Healers on Healing*, "Unless the possibility of something good is attached to the prospect of treatment, the environment of treatment may be impaired....If a patient comes away from a diagnosis in a state of emotional devastation, the stage may be set for rapid advance of the disease."

If someone is presented with a negative prognosis, it is important not to lose hope. A negative prognosis can serve as a challenge to mobilize a person's will to live and inner healing resources. No one can foresee the outcome of an illness with absolute certainty. A condition that appears hopeless from one point of view may appear hopeful from another. There are numerous stories of exceptional patients who changed their diet and lifestyle and went on to completely recover despite a negative prognosis. Accounts such as these prove that when provided with a restorative diet and supportive environment, human beings have the inner resources to overcome practically any illness.

Meditation and Visualization

Quieting the mind through meditation helps dissolve negative thoughts that interfere with the process of healing. Negative thoughts and emotions disturb the smooth flow of healing energy in the chakras, meridians, and cells. Clearing the mind of unnecessary or unhelpful thoughts allows healing energy to flow smoothly. Meditation, including the simple regulation of breathing, can thus be a powerful tool in healing. Meditation is now being used by doctors to train patients to relax the tone of autonomic nerves, lower blood pressure, and relieve stress on the heart and other internal organs. Persons who are skilled at meditation have demonstrated the ability to consciously control their digestive, respiratory, and circulatory functions. A variety of conditions are now linked to over-stimulation of the sympathetic branch of the autonomic nervous system, including high blood pressure, irregular heart beating, and various digestive disorders. By calming and relaxing this system, regular meditation can help normalize these and other conditions.

To practice the most basic form of meditation, do the following:

1. Find a quiet place and sit in a relaxed and comfortable position. Yoga practices usually recommend the half-lotus position, but this can induce the tendency to hunch over. To keep the spine straight while sitting in this position, you can sit on a pillow or cushion. An even better way of sitting is to sit on the heels; that is, with the feet tucked under the legs so that the arches of the feet form a rounded place to sit in. The big toes should hold each other: one on top of the other, and if your condition is good, you can sit like this for hours. When you are tired, just reverse the position of your toes.

   The reason why some people cannot sit this way is because they do not eat well; for example, too much animal food, fruit, or baked flour products, or too much eating in general. If the joints are stiff or swollen, it is difficult to sit in this manner. As one's condition improves through proper eating and physical activity, it becomes easier and more comfortable to sit this way. In the meantime, if you are not comfortable sitting on the floor, sitting in a chair is also fine.

2. The most effective and relaxing meditation is done when your posture is straight but relaxed. To straighten your posture, raise your arms up toward the ceiling and hold them there for a few moments. Then tilt your head so that you are looking up. Keep your head in this position for several seconds, and then lower your arms to their normal position at your side. Return your head to normal a moment later. This simple stretching exercise straightens the spine and allows energy from heaven and earth to flow smoothly through the body. Each of these steps can be done as a continuous sequence and the entire procedure can be repeated several times.

3. With your spine straight and your shoulders and elbows relaxed, place your hands in your lap with the palms facing up. Place your left hand, which corresponds to heaven, on top of your right, which corresponds to the earth. Lift your thumbs upward and touch the tips of both thumbs together, forming an arc, or bridge. Your thumbs and index fingers should generally form a circle. This position creates unity and harmony between the left and right sides of the body, and between the flow of heaven's and earth's forces.

4. Close your eyes and begin to breathe naturally and quietly. Breathe in a normal, relaxed manner. After making your breathing calm and quiet, begin to breathe deeply, centering your breath in the lower abdomen, or hara. As you breathe in, let your abdomen expand; and as you breathe out, let it contract.

5. While you are breathing in this manner, let your mind become quiet, relaxed, and free of distracting thoughts or images. Do not try to force distracting thoughts to go away but simply let them dissolve. It may help to concentrate on

your breathing. Sit this way for several minutes, breathing naturally and keeping your mind still and quiet. Let your body relax.

6. To complete your meditation, slowly open your eyes and let your breathing return to normal. Then bring your consciousness back to a normal waking state.

Once the mind has been cleared of unnecessary distractions, it is much easier to practice positive visualization, or creative imaging. Peaceful, positive images of health or tranquil images of nature are more conducive to healing than are images that focus on sickness or struggle. Visualizing illness as an enemy that you are struggling against creates stress and anxiety that interferes with the harmonious flow of energy throughout the body.

To practice visualization, begin to meditate as above, and when you reach step four, form an image of yourself as a healthy and happy person. Do not dwell on illness or imperfections, but see yourself as you would like to be. Let your image develop for several minutes then return your mind to a peaceful, quiet state. This practice can be done as often as necessary to reduce stress and inspire hope for the future. As you continue practicing, start to see your daily life as the process through which you actualize this positive, healthy image of yourself.

Visualizing Healing Energy

Another type of visualization can be done in which you create an image of the healing energy that flows through the chakras, meridians, and cells. To visualize healing energy in the chakras, begin with the standard meditation described above. When you reach step four, and your mind is quiet and tranquil, focus your awareness at the top of the head where the seventh, or crown chakra is located. If you detect tightness, blockage, or tension in this region, let it dissolve and melt away. Keep your awareness focused here for a minute or two, and then move it down to the sixth, or midbrain chakra in the region behind the eyes. If you feel tension or tightness anywhere in the head, allow it to relax and dissolve. Center your awareness here for a minute or two and then proceed to center of the throat, where the fifth chakra is located. Try to relax tension in the throat and lower jaw, and after a minute or two, proceed to the heart chakra in the center of the chest. Become aware of your heartbeat and the energy flowing behind and through it and let that energy flow throughout the chest, dissolving and melting any tightness or tension. Hold your attention here for a minute or two, and then proceed to the stomach chakra in the center of the solar plexus, the hara chakra in the center of the abdomen, and the first, or base chakra at the base of the spine. As you focus attention in each chakra, try to relax tension in the corresponding region of the body.

Now that your body is relaxed and energized, repeat the exercise, this time, with the added dimension of active visualization. As your consciousness merges with each chakra, visualize energy—in the form of shining white light—radiating from the chakra to the part of the body surrounding it. Start with the crown chakra and proceed downward, visualizing the energy in each chakra for about a minute or two before proceeding to the next. Visualize each chakra as a miniature sun radiating light. After you have visualized energy in all seven chakras, visualize your entire body as an interconnected web of light and energy. Allow energy to circulate without interference from the central chakra line out to the periphery of the body, so that each cell is bathed in and illuminated by light, and then from the periphery of the body back to the centrally located chakras. Keep your breathing natural and relaxed. After several minutes, your entire body should be completely relaxed, yet fully charged with energy. Then let the visualization gradually subside and allow your consciousness to return to its normal waking state. Slowly open your eyes and return to normal.

To focus chakra energy in a specific location, such as a part of the body where you feel pain, practice the visualization described above. Once you have visualized energy flowing throughout the body, start to visualize light and energy streaming into the part of the body you wish to heal. At the same time, use your consciousness to relax the area and dissolve any tension that might be present. Visualize energy flowing into the region from the entire body, and then back again. Let stagnated energy in the region melt into the general circulation of energy as a whole. When the area starts to feel light and energized, let the visualization subside and your consciousness return to normal.

Natural Meditation

Nature is the source of our self-healing abilities. Meditating on such natural phenomena as the rising sun, the ocean, mountains, a beautiful lake or a flowing stream, or the moon and stars helps us reconnect with the source of healing. Like positive imaging, it inspires confidence and hope. Natural meditation relaxes the body and mind and helps us put our problems in perspective and realize that they are small and ephemeral in comparison to the eternal cycles of nature. It releases us from the one-sided preoccupation with our small selves.

In a study conducted by researchers at the University of Delaware, visual contact with nature was found to accelerate healing. Patients recovering from gallbladder surgery were divided into two groups: one in hospital rooms with a window that faced a stand of trees, and the other with a window that faced a brick wall. The group with the view of the trees experienced a smoother recovery, with fewer postoperative complications, less pain medication, and fewer days in the hospital.

Natural meditation can be practiced in several ways. The passive form consists of simply being mindful of the natural world while engaged in day to day activities. Try to become conscious of nature while at home or at the office, or while riding in a car or walking down the street. Taking time every day for a brisk, half-hour walk is especially helpful, as walking offers an opportunity to contact nature while experiencing the benefits of physical activity. The active form of natural meditation involves actually going outside and focusing your attention on some natural object or scene, such as a pond, mountains, a cluster of trees, a waterfall, the moon or stars. You can simply sit with a quiet mind and admire the object or scene for several minutes, or can practice a more formal routine.

To practice formal meditation, do the basic meditation described above, and when you reach step four, open your eyes and contemplate the natural object or scene. Try to feel at one with it. After several minutes, close your eyes, sit quietly for a few seconds, and return to normal. Breathe naturally and peacefully while you are meditating. Natural meditation has a calming and tranquilizing effect on the mind and body, allows healing energy to flow smoothly, and dissolves stress produced by living and working in the artificial, mechanical environments of modern civilization.

Diet and Consciousness

The brain and nervous system are especially sensitive to the biochemical environment of the body. Chemical changes in the brain's blood supply, whether caused by alcohol, drugs, or daily foods, produce corresponding changes in mood, thinking, and behavior.

Daily foods influence the secretion of hormones, and these in turn affect the brain and nervous system. In a study conducted by medical researchers at Yale, the intake of refined sugar was found to dramatically increase blood levels of adrenaline in children. In children who were tested after being given an amount of sugar equal to two cupcakes, levels of adrenaline increased ten times. Adrenaline, secreted by the adrenal glands during times of stress, triggers the so-called "fight or flight" response, with such effects as a rapid heartbeat, quick shallow breathing, and nervousness. Increased adrenaline levels could also lead to anxiety and difficulty in concentrating. Parents have often noticed that children display hyperactive, aggressive, or erratic behavior following the intake of sugary foods, and this study offers a possible biochemical explanation for this reaction.

Diet also affects the concentration of neurotransmitters in the brain, and hence our perceptions and behavior. Eggs and other animal proteins increase the levels of acetylcholine in the brain, while foods such as whole grains, beans, and vegetables rich in complex carbohydrates increase the brain's supply of serotonin, a neurotransmitter believed to induce calm and relaxed mental states. That may help explain why persons who consume grains and vegetables and little animal food seem calm and even-tempered in comparison to heavy meat eaters. On the other hand, the low levels of serotonin that result from a diet high in animal foods, may contribute to impulsive behavior. In studies of prison inmates conducted in Finland, those with the most impulsive behavior patterns were found to have the lowest levels of metabolized serotonin in the spinal fluid when compared to non-impulsive prisoners and controls. The impulsive inmates were also found to have low blood sugar levels. The researchers found that 81 percent of repeat offenders had abnormally low blood sugar levels. Low levels of serotonin, together with low levels of blood sugar, characterized 84 percent of the repeat offenders studied.

Chronic low blood sugar, or hypoglycemia, is related to the health and functioning of the pancreas. The hard fats contained in animal foods, especially those in chicken, cheese, eggs, and shellfish, accumulate in the pancreas, making the organ hard and tight. The pancreas secretes insulin and anti-insulin (glucagon). Insulin keeps the blood sugar level down, while anti-insulin causes it to rise.

When blood sugar rises, insulin is automatically secreted in order to bring it down. If, for example, someone eats refined sugar, ice cream, fruit, chocolate, or other simple sugars that are rapidly absorbed, the amount of sugar in the blood quickly goes up and insulin is secreted. Insulin causes sugar to enter the cells and be oxidized, thus lowering the level of glucose in the blood. As the blood sugar level drops, the pancreas secretes anti-insulin to keep it from dropping too far. If we are healthy, these pancreatic hormones act to maintain the proper level of sugar in the blood.

However, when the pancreas becomes overly tight and hard fats develop within it, it is no longer able to secrete anti-insulin properly. The result is hypoglycemia. This condition is caused by the overconsumption of animal food and produces cravings for sugar, alcohol, or strong sweets. When blood sugar dips below normal, the person will seek to raise it usually by taking in some form of simple sugar. He may reach for a chocolate bar, a soft drink, or coffee with sugar, or in some cases, alcohol, in an attempt to make balance.

The brain is the largest consumer of glucose in the body, and low blood sugar levels have an acute effect on it, and hence on moods and emotions. Low blood sugar elicits a shutting down of brain functions that are biologically less essential to conserve the more essential, mechanical functions necessary for survival. The less essential is the cerebellum, which controls the refined, higher levels of human consciousness including aesthetic perception and reasoning ability. With these functions impaired, a person tends to revert to irrational behavior tendencies governed by the cerebrum, which regulates breathing, heart action, and muscular activity in the "fight or flight" category, also known as the panic response. As the higher reasoning centers shut down, a person will experience a feeling of being trapped or confined by circumstances, along with anxiety and depression at the perceived inability to change one's situation for the better. These mental states interfere with a person's self-healing abilities.

Dissolving Energy Blocks

As long as we are alive, heaven's and earth's forces are constantly charging the primary channel that runs slightly in front of the spine through the length of the body. The life energy running through this central meridian is distributed throughout the body, creating the rhythm of the cardiac muscles, the peristaltic action of the digestive organs, the high-speed firing of nerve impulses, the contraction and extension of the muscles, the hormone secretion of the endocrine glands, and all of the body's movements. This is not a steady stream of energy, but an alternating current of heaven's and earth's forces flowing straight through the body and uniting its functions in an unbroken, pulsating rhythm of life. When the primary channel is clear, you automatically feel at one with the environment, physically, mentally, and spiritually. Images arising in the midbrain are transmitted directly to the cells through the network of meridians and meridian branches. However, if the muscles, tissues, and internal organs become hard and rigid, and lose their normal flexibility, conductivity is reduced and the flow of energy through these pathways is impeded. Patterns of tension can become frozen, distorting the posture and causing the person to sit, stand, and move in patterns of tightness and rigidity. Rather than being discharged and let go, negative thoughts and emotions are internalized and held onto, and remain in the body in the form of frozen energy patterns.

The ability to express oneself freely and honestly is a sign that energy is flowing actively through the body, while the inability to express oneself is a sign that the flow of energy is blocked by our physical condition. Numerous studies have pointed to a connection between repressed emotions and disease. Many doctors have noted that lung cancer patients have the tendency to suppress their emotions, while studies of cancer patients have shown that long-term survivors tended to express negative emotions while those who did not survive tended to hold their emotions in. Emotions are a vehicle for discharging excess that contributes to illness. Crying, for example, is a way of eliminating excessive factors from the body. Emotional tears contain more protein than tears caused by irritants such as dust.

Hardening along the primary channel, in the chakras, or along the meridians is the primary impediment to the free flow of energy throughout the body. When the channels of transmission are blocked, we are less able to use our consciousness to influence our health in a positive way. Activities such as positive imaging and creative visualization are less effective than they could be.

An unbalanced diet is the main cause of the rigidity that interferes with the flow of energy. Among modern foods, those containing hard saturated fat are the leading contributors to hardening along the primary channel, in the chakras, and along the meridians. Fat accounts for as much as 42 percent of the daily diet of people in the United States, according to some surveys, and a large part is eaten in the form of saturated fat. The relationship between a high-fat diet and heart disease and cancer is becoming widely known, and most nutritionists and public health organizations agree with the macrobiotic suggestion that the amount of fat in the modern diet be substantially reduced.

Animal foods are the only source of cholesterol and the chief source of saturated fat in the modern diet. When eaten excessively, animal foods cause fat and cholesterol to accumulate internally. When this happens in the arteries and blood vessels, the result is heart disease. But beyond affecting the blood vessels, saturated fats also produce varying degrees of hardening throughout the body, including the skin, internal organs, chakras, and along the meridians and primary channel. When meat, eggs, butter, poultry, and cheese are eaten regularly, the accumulation of fat and cholesterol causes the body to become rigid and inflexible. Saturated fat also causes the skin to become hard, tough, and insensitive. The flow of energy through the primary channel, chakras, and meridians is considerably weakened as a result.

The meridians run just below the skin, and differentiate into numerous tiny branches that connect to the cells. Whether or not energy flows smoothly through these pathways depends on the condition of the skin, including the minute blood capillaries that supply it with oxygen and nutrients. Blood vessels, skin, and other tissues are composed of collagen and elastin, the primary proteins that make up the body's connective tissues. Elastin provides flexibility, softness, and elasticity to the skin, while collagen imparts the toughness that holds it together. When the diet is high in animal foods that contain saturated fat, a variety of things happen to these tissues. When eaten excessively, high-fat foods cause the ratio of collagen and elastin to gradually shift. A diet high in animal foods causes a gradual depletion of elastin, so that collagen becomes prevalent. As a result, the skin loses its normal flexibility and eventually becomes hard and inelastic.

Overconsumption of fat also accelerates a process known as "cross-linking," in which collagen changes from a soluble to insoluble form. In children, for example, collagen exists in a flexible form and is made up of short cables that are distinct from one another. The breakdown of fats releases free radicals, which are highly volatile, destructive bits of matter that damage tissues. These stray molecules wedge between the collagen cables, causing them to gradually clump together and become knotted with tough fibers. The result is stiffening, hardening, and loss of elasticity in the skin and other tissues throughout the body. In this condition, energy does not flow smoothly throughout the body.

Daily foods affect more than just the transmission of energy through the chakras and meridians. They also influence the thoughts and images that arise in the brain. When our condition is healthy and balanced, energy flows actively through the body. We feel connected to nature and other people, and this sense of connectedness inspires confidence and hope. On the other hand, if our condition becomes rigid and inflexible, due to the overconsumption of animal foods, conductivity to heaven's and earth's forces diminishes. We begin to feel cut off from nature and other people, and experience a false sense of isolation. Our existence becomes increasingly self-centered.

Nature is the source of life, and the force behind all healing, and if we lose contact with it, we confine ourselves to a diminishing range of possibilities. We become increasingly isolated, anxious, and alone. In this condition, it is difficult to form clear, positive, and optimistic mental images, and as a result, we are more likely to be overwhelmed by circumstances and succumb to negative emotions. It is also difficult to form meaningful and long-lasting bonds with other people. Social and family ties are easily disrupted, with direct consequences for one's health. It is widely known that persons with disrupted or weakened social and family ties have an increased susceptibility to disease. This phenomenon is described by Robert Ornstein, Ph.D., and David Sobel, M.D., in *The Healing Brain*:

> People who are single, separated, divorced, or widowed are two or three times more likely to die than their married peers. They also wind up in the hospital for mental disorders

five to ten times as frequently. Whether we look at heart disease, cancer, depression, tuberculosis, arthritis, or problems during pregnancy, the occurrence of disease is higher in those with weakened social connectedness.

A depressed or agitated mental state makes it difficult to quiet the mind through meditation, and sends a variety of conflicting signals to the body. Rather than being calm and in control, a person may swing back and forth between the extremes of powerlessness and resignation on one hand, and anger and struggle on the other. This condition is made worse by hypoglycemia, which results from overconsuming the types of foods that cause stagnation in the body's energy flow. Hypoglycemia leads to bouts of depression and self-doubt that undermine the process of healing, and can reduce the decision-making process to a series of "fight or flight" or panic responses.

Without a change in diet, activities such as positive mental imaging, meditation, and visualization are of limited benefit. In some cases, they may be helpful in furthering the process of healing, or in temporarily reducing symptoms, but without more fundamental change, the illness often returns or reappears in another form. By themselves, these practices do not fully address the underlying biological imbalances that produce sickness. Mind and body are one, and for fundamental healing to occur, we need to consider both.

Holistic Healing

Traditional healing systems aimed at dissolving energy blockages. Together with avoiding high-fat animal foods and eating a naturally balanced diet, two other practices can also be used to restore active energy flow. The first is simply to be active physically, mentally, and spiritually. Anything is fine—walking every day, cleaning floors, cooking, washing dishes, studying, meditating, exercising, or practicing visualization. It is important to be regularly active in all three of these ways; otherwise you will favor one chakra or another, one way of thinking or another, and fail to achieve harmony or balance as a whole.

The second way is to practice a simple form of chanting to energize your chakras, meridians, and primary channel. Sound is a form of vibration, and when practiced correctly, stimulates these energy pathways and helps dissolve stagnation. The sound "AAA" (pronounced "AHH") vibrates the lower body in the area of the stomach and intestines. The sound "UUU" vibrates in the the heart, lungs, and middle region of the body, and the sound "MMM" vibrates in the throat and head. When you make these sounds together, "A-U-M," repeating this perhaps ten or twenty times each day, you can help clear the primary channel, chakras, and meridians of blockage and stagnation. To practice this simple chant, sit as described above with your spine straight and body relaxed. Close your eyes and let your mind become quiet. Then breathe in and make the sound "A-U-M," long and slowly with a deep exhalation. After repeating the sound ten or twenty times, sit with your eyes closed for about one minute more. Then slowly open your eyes and resume your activities.

Holistic healing considers mind and body as one. Evidence is accumulating that the combination of a naturally balanced diet, moderate exercise, and mental relaxation may not only prevent, but also help reverse, degenerative illness. Today it is common knowledge that diet can play a significant role in preventing cancer, heart disease, and other degenerative conditions. Numerous medical studies linking the modern high-fat, high-cholesterol diet with breast, colon, prostate, ovarian, and other cancers have provided support to the macrobiotic dietary and lifestyle approach. In the book *Cancer-Free: 30 Who Triumphed Over Cancer Naturally* (Tokyo and New York: Japan Publications, Inc., 1992), the East West Foundation presents further evidence that a naturally balanced macrobiotic diet, in combination with a positive mental attitude, moderate exercise, and other natural living practices, can dramatically and positively influence the outcome of already existing cancers.

The book contains personal accounts of thirty people from many walks of life—including housewives, business executives, a medical doctor, a registered nurse, an autoworker, a stockbroker, a nutritionist, a senior administrator for the U.N.—who recovered from a wide variety of malignancies, including breast cancer, colon cancer, stomach cancer, pancreatic cancer, lung cancer, ovarian cancer, uterine cancer, prostate cancer, bone cancer, brain tumor, melanoma, leukemia, and Hodgkin's disease. Besides personal narratives, the study includes several medically documented cases of terminal cancer remission by Vivien Newbold, M.D., a physician practicing in Philadelphia.

The separation of the individual from the process of healing has not served us well. The rise of chronic diseases in the twentieth century—including heart disease, cancer, AIDS and immune deficiencies, diabetes, and arthritis—has revealed the limits of the model of health and healing based on the artificial separation of body and mind.

Catastrophic conditions exact a high price from our society, both in terms of personal suffering and economic impact. Staggering increases in medical costs are leading modern society toward bankruptcy. Driven by the decline in personal health, medical costs currently consume 12 percent of the Gross National Product in the United States, double the amount spent for national defense. Medical costs are increasing at such a rate that, unless this trend is reversed, they will consume the entire GNP by the middle of the next century. However, this trend will not reverse unless we shift the emphasis of the modern health care system from treating disease to preventing it, and begin incorporating things such as balanced natural diet, mental relaxation, and stress reduction into our approach to treating chronic illness. Individual actions are far more important than medical intervention in avoiding degenerative diseases, and play a vital role in healing and regeneration. The body is not a machine with replaceable parts but an integrated whole with both tangible and intangible dimensions. It is therefore time to reposition the individual at the center of the healing process, and reunite mind, body, and spirit in our approach to health and healing.

Spiritual Dimensions of Healing

Holistic healing considers not only the visible, physical aspects of our being, but also the invisible, spiritual aspects. Human beings are made up of more than just flesh and bones. The human body is actually composed of seven layers, some of which are vibrational, others of which are material. Brown rice also has seven layers, making it a complete spiral. The physical body is made up of three spirally formed systems: the digestive-respiratory system, the nervous system, and the circulatory-excretory system. The earth is formed in a similar way, with an inner layer, or crust, composed of minerals, a middle layer comprised of water, and an outer layer made up of air. The crust is very yang, air is very yin, and water is in-between. The watery environment lies in-between the states of gas and solidity, and is where life begins. Our digestive system is yin—hollow and expanded, our brain and nervous system are yang—compact and solid, and our circulatory system is in-between. In the body, the circulation of fluid is similar to the water on the surface of the earth.

Our bodies are not limited to their physical aspects only, but are composed of the following seven layers in a huge spiral that traverses both the physical and vibrational worlds:

Material or Elemental Body The innermost layer of the body includes the compact bones and is composed of elements in the form of minerals, liquids, and gases. It is responsible for involuntary, mechanical responses, such as those occurring in the case of shock, without the involvement of conscious awareness.

Protoplasmic Body The second layer of the body is composed of protoplasm, and takes a jelly-like form. It is not exclusively solid, liquid, or gas, but very mixed up. Most cells are made up of protoplasm. The protoplasmic body is the source of sensory awareness.

Plasmic Body The third layer of the body envelops the first two and is the source of emotions and feelings. It is sometimes referred to as the astral body or aura, and generates feelings of temperature, pressure, and heat. The plasmic body includes the energy flowing through the chakras and meridians, and like a ghost, separates from the physical body at death. It includes the heat and caloric energy generated by the body, and is governed by a subtle form of electricity.

The physical body is composed of levels one and two. Modern nutrition is based on a materialistic view and deals only with the needs of the first two bodies. It does not consider the third body or those beyond it. The concept of death exists only for people who assume that existence is limited to the physical world. When we separate from the first and second bodies at death, some of our activities cease. However, five additional layers are still there, and in certain respects, life after death is more active than life in the physical world.

Vibrating Body When plasma is active, it produces vibrations. The fourth layer of the body is composed of vibrations and minute pre-electronic particles. We cannot see the vibrating body but we can feel it. It is the source of our intellectual and social consciousness, and is governed by the force of magnetism. Communication begins with the third and fourth bodies, while on levels one and two, there is only individual feeling. The vibrating body is sometimes referred to as the soul.

Electromagnetic Waving Body The fifth layer of the body is composed of subtle refined waves. With it we are able to communicate across great distances, even thousands of miles, through extrasensory perception and telepathy. You activate this body when you have a certain feeling about a friend or relative far away, or a premonition about something in the future.

Each layer of our spiritual body corresponds to a color. Noncolor includes all colors, just as silence represents the complete harmony of all sounds.

When waves move at high speeds, they cluster and appear as particles, which we may refer to as *spiritual particles*. Each particle is nothing but weight. The realm of these particles is where our understanding begins. The formation of images occurs here; mental pictures and imagination arise from this layer of the body. If your health is good, these images are true; if not,

Relationship of Spiritual Constitution and Colors

Body	Level of Consciousness	Color
Material	Mechanical	Red
Protoplasmic	Sensory	Orange
Plasmic	Emotional	Yellow/gold
Vibrating	Intellectual	Green
Electromagnetic	Social	Blue
Ultrawaving	Spiritual	Violet
Universal	Cosmic	Non-color

they are fantasies. The electromagnetic waving body is sometimes referred to as the spirit.

Ultrawaving Body The ultrawaving body is difficult to perceive. It encompasses the world of yin and yang, or pure expanding and contracting motion. It is the origin of all forms of consciousness. Various forms of meditation are aimed at developing this layer of the body. In metaphysical terms, the ultrawaving body is referred to as pure consciousness or spirit.

Universal, Infinitely Expanding Body All of us are within the infinitely expanding, universal spirit. The infinite universe exists everywhere, throughout all time, and is endlessly differentiating, developing, changing, and producing. It is the source of everything. In the physical world, the universal body appears as nothing. In religious terms, it is referred to as God, Brahman, or nirvana. It is the source of universal, all-embracing consciousness, which we perceive as a feeling of oneness or intuition. Here there is no time nor space, but infinite depth, endless time, and boundless space. It is the state of pure being.

Time and space are a small part of infinity. They are, in reality, the product of our relative imagination. Infinity has no time and no space, although it is the source of all time and all space. Our experience of time and space begins at the fifth layer of the body. All human desires arise from the perception of time and space. Desire, attachment, and delusion increase in strength as the levels develop inward toward the physical body.

After death, we shed these bodies one by one until we return to the infinite universe itself. This process of transformation is like that in which a silkworm enters its cocoon and emerges as moth. At birth, we emerge from the watery environment of the womb, and begin to breathe air and eat foods from the earth. Our body is made of elements and protoplasm. Then, in the next stage, the higher, vibrational bodies withdraw from the physical body at death and continue living within the world of vibrations or energy. In time, we change into each of these higher layers, becoming freer and freer, until ultimately we become the seventh body itself. Then we are completely free; omnipresent, omnipotent, God itself.

The amount of time spent on each of these levels varies greatly from person to person. Some people spend a long time on a particular level, others rapidly change levels. At the highest level, time disappears, and we exist only in the present.

In the plasmic body, love is the highest emotional experience. The plasmic body is influenced greatly by what we eat. Therefore, our destiny in the next life, in which our primary body is the plasmic body, is determined by our daily eating, and the extent to which we develop such qualities as love, sympathy, and understanding. An egocentric, uncaring person will have a narrow, dark existence in the next world. A person who sacrifices for others, while eating well and maintaining good physical and mental health, will be happy in the next life. Each of our lives is preparation for the next. Whether your next life is free and happy or narrow and dark depends on your state of health and whether or not you develop love and compassion for others.

When your physical body is disturbed as the result of illness, so are your higher bodies. They do not synchronize properly with your physical body or with each other. If our health is poor, our mind, body, and spirit do not harmonize properly. On the other hand, if each of the body's cells is synchronized with the seventh body, that person has what we might call absolute intuition.

Before we are born, our space in the womb is small. After birth, we have the whole earth. In the next life, our space expands to include the whole solar system and galaxy. The fourth body's field of activity covers the whole universe, while the fifth, sixth, and seventh bodies range far beyond this universe. These are the dimensions of the spiritual world. After ten, twenty, or thirty years of living macrobiotically, you start to know more of these invisible worlds. As your insight and understanding increase, you begin to sense the presence of these worlds and live according to this awareness.

The earth is small in comparison to the dimensions of space that we experience during our life journey from infinity to this world and back again. Being healthy means that we consider not only our life in this world, but also in the worlds to come. To do this, we need to carefully consider what it is we want to do in this life, including how we wish to eat, and how to develop love, understanding, and compassion.

Nourishing the Spirit

The material body is composed of solid matter, including iron and other minerals, and produces mechanical consciousness. The second body is made up of protoplasm in the form of expanding and contracting cells, and produces sensory awareness. The third, plasmic or bioplasmic body is composed of energy, calories, and heat. It produces emotions, including those of love and hate, like and dislike. Palm healing, which we discuss in the next chapter, is based on the active use of this energy. On the fourth level, the vibrating body, we use our intellectual and social understanding, and make judgments based on whether we think something is reasonable or unreasonable, correct or incorrect. With the fifth, electromagnetic waving body, we recognize the basic force of the universe, that of attraction and repulsion. Philosophical consciousness, including basic awareness of universal truth, begins at this level. The sixth, ultrawaving body, produces such attributes as gratitude, affirmation, appreciation, and the sense of wonder and marvel. The universal body is the source of cosmic consciousness. It is the world of God or wholeness.

These seven bodies are constantly receiving nourishment from the environment. When you were in your mother's womb, you were nourished by her bloodstream, which is rich in iron and other minerals. Using these elements, you formed your material and protoplasmic bodies. After birth, these bodies are nourished by the products of the earth, including minerals, proteins, and carbohydrates, together with oxygen from the atmosphere. We also take vibrations from the air, including light through the eyes, and begin receiving invisible vibrations through the so-called *third eye*, the place on the forehead that corresponds to the midbrain chakra. These vibrational foods provide nourishment for our higher bodies.

The central core of the earth is composed of iron and other metals. The earth's crust is made up of minerals and heavy liquid. It contains many chemical compounds, but its main substance is carbon. The atmosphere is composed of gases such as nitrogen, oxygen, and carbon dioxide. At the outermost periphery of the atmosphere we find hydrogen, and beyond that, free electrons and preatomic particles. Our planetary environment is surrounded by vibrations, including those produced by the sun and stars, along with electromagnetic energy, ultrawaving energy, cosmic rays, and ultimately, the primary expanding force of the universe itself.

Every few hours we nourish ourselves with the material foods of the earth; we take air more frequently, and are constantly taking in vibrations. The world of vibrations is more universal and all-encompassing than the physical world of the earth. Vibrations exist everywhere, and we have no need to store them inside the body. Nor do we need to transport them. When we die, we no longer eat physical food, but are nourished entirely by vibrations. In the seventh world, food and you become one; there is no longer a distinction between self and nourishment.

In order to be healthy in this world, it is essential to be properly nourished in the womb. The mother's diet, in addition to her thoughts and activity, plays a decisive role in determining whether or not her baby will have a healthy and happy life. In a similar way, how we eat in this life has a profound influence on our life in the next world. The plasmic body produces emotions and feelings, and these determine the kind of life we experience in the next world. If we develop genuine love for others in this lifetime, when we are reborn in the next life, we enter the higher and more refined realms of the plasmic world. When we go on to the next level of the spiritual world, the kind of life we experience in those dimensions depends upon our development in the plasmic world. Each world is preparation for the next.

Reincarnation takes place from within the plasmic world. The astral, or plasmic world includes the surface of the earth and occupies the lower realms of the spiritual world. That world is also the source of ghosts. If you have strong emotional attachment to your human experience, your plasmic body will again incarnate materially. In some cases, these attachments are so strong that they cause the person's plasmic body to remain in the general vicinity of his earthly life, or to attach to a husband, wife, child, relative, or close associate. However, if your consciousness is thoroughly developed at death and you have no attachment—meaning that your plasmic body becomes light and refined, while assuming a wave-like form—then rather than being born again in physical form, you proceed to the higher realms of the spiritual world.

In this world, we communicate through words. In the next world, we communicate via thought; in the world that follows, through images; then through feelings that travel instantaneously throughout the universe. Ultimately, thought and action become one. The distinction between thought, feeling, and action disappears entirely. On that level, whatever we imagine is realized as soon as the image begins to take form.

It is easier to recall our origin in the spiritual world than it is to remember past lives on earth. Children grow rapidly and live mostly in the present; it is usually difficult for them to remember events of the week before. Similarly, we usually cannot remember our life in the womb, because, at these stages of life, change is rapid. But if we go further back, we penetrate to the source of this universe—the world of vibrations or waves—where things do not change form as rapidly as they do in the material world.

In higher worlds things become more constant, and we can recall these invisible worlds even though we are living in the physical world where change is dynamic and rapid.

Subconsciously you may be thinking that your life is ephemeral and that someday you will die. But in another part of your consciousness, you feel that your life is eternal and continues after death. Those feelings arise when your body synchronizes with the spiritual world, enabling you to understand and remember your endless life. The aim of holistic, macrobiotic healing is to accelerate the growth of consciousness toward universal, all-embracing love. Then, when you die, your next life is much happier and easier. You have a good foundation from your previous life, and if you develop enough, you can go on to higher levels without coming back to the earth. As you continue on your spiritual journey, your playground becomes larger and larger, embracing the solar system, Milky Way galaxy, then the universe; and ultimately far beyond the visible, detectable universe. Through macrobiotic living, you can develop a refined spiritual nature. As your sensitivity returns, your memory of these invisible worlds will become clearer, and you start to understand them in a practical, non-mystical way.

3
Healing with Energy

Although the concept of Ki, or energy, is not generally found in Western society, it is a basic concept in Oriental medicine. The understanding and use of Ki is inseparable from Eastern medicine, religion, and philosophy, and the entire way of life in the Orient. Although it is expressed in different terms in each culture, it is common to all traditional societies in the East.

Ancient philosopher-healers saw life in terms of Ki. Their understanding of life was non-material. By contrast, most people today, including those in science and medicine, equate life with the world of matter. Modern understanding tends to be limited to the material world, and that is why the concept of energy or spirit is difficult for modern people to grasp.

In Chapter 1 we saw how the spiral of materialization describes movement from the infinitely large to the infinitely small, including the appearance of humanity. Out of the centrifugal motion of infinity, which means infinite motion at infinite speed, two waves of motion collide, creating a centripetal, inward-moving spiral. Polarity, or yin and yang, are then produced, leading to the appearance of vibrations, preatomic particles, elements, the world of vegetables, and finally to the world of animals, including our own species.

Human beings are the end point of this spiral, through which the invisible becomes visible, and the infinite takes tangible form. The fully developed spirals that result in the appearance of human beings take billions of years to reach maturity. From here, we begin to journey in the opposite direction; we return to infinity by way of an expanding, centrifugal spiral, in which our consciousness develops to where it can embrace the whole universe.

Traditional philosopher-healers explained the world of matter, including the human body, in terms of non-material energy. They understood that energy, or non-matter, exists within the world of matter. Matter arises from non-matter, as a transformed version of it; like a ghost that seems to appear out of nowhere and then vanishes. The origin of both matter and non-matter is the invisible vibrational force, which is referred to as energy in modern science. But when traditional healers spoke of energy, they were not talking only about detectable energy, such as heat, light, or electromagnetic waves. Entire universes of energy exist beyond the realm of our senses and detecting machines. And all of this, the visible and non-visible, the physical and non-physical, ancient philosopher-healers called Ki.

If you imagine that Ki is only detectable energy, you are only partly right. And if you think Ki is electromagnetic energy, you are again only partly right. Ki is found from the infinitesimally shortest wave to the infinitely longest wave; from the most rapidly moving waves to the slowest. It includes all of this, everything. Ki is covering the entire universe. It is a universal phenomenon.

Health depends on maintaining dynamic balance between the energy of the body, or internal Ki, and the energy of the environment, or external Ki. Below we examine the relationship between the two, as well as the role of our diet, daily activity, and way of thinking in creating harmony between them.

Our Internal and External Body

Long ago, the earth was covered with heavy gases like methane, ammonia, and water vapor, all of which are heavier than the current atmosphere of oxygen and nitrogen. Life began under these conditions. The first organization of organic compounds was made almost four billion years ago, and the most primary single-celled life forms appeared about 3.2 billion years ago as the atmosphere became clearer. At that time, the earth was becoming dense and compact, evolving toward its present form from a condition resembling that of Jupiter.

The atmosphere has become clearer up to the present, and its color has gradually changed from red to blue. Because the atmosphere changed from yang (dense and reddish color) to yin (clear and blue), there may have been a yellow atmosphere at some time in the past. Meanwhile, animal and vegetable life developed from a single cell into complex levels of multi-cellular organization. Tissues, organs, and complex systems became more specialized until humanity, with trillions of cells, appeared.

When the sky is cloudy and thick, as it was in the ancient past, it is impossible to see any stars or even the sun, even though the earth is still receiving cosmic radiation. As time went by, the sun and moon, plus hundreds, then thousands, and finally millions of stars became visible. Our body is always balancing with the environment. The influences received from the universe produce changes in the structure of biological life, including the type and number of cells. If the environment is expanded, more complicated bodies appear to make balance.

Single-celled life started under a yang, heavy atmosphere when only the sun was visible; the first multi-cellular organisms developed at a time when the earth was receiving influence from the sun, moon, Venus, and some bright stars nearby. Because the atmosphere is clearer now, we are receiving influence from many distant stars, and biological bodies developed billions of cells in response. When millions of stars became visible, millions of cells appeared to make balance.

Each cell in the human body has a spiral character with a nucleus at the center. In the center of the nucleus is DNA, which takes the form of a double-helix that reflects the spiral pattern found throughout nature. Each cell corresponds to and makes balance with one of the trillions of suns in the universe, the vibrations of which are being received at the surface of the earth. Many of these stars are not detectable with telescopes.

When the first one-celled amoeba appeared on earth, only the sun's influence was felt. Single-celled animals make balance with the sun, which is yang. They require dark, humid surroundings (yin) that correspond to the heavy atmosphere in which they developed. In a similar way our brain has billions of cells that correspond to the billions of stars in the Milky Way galaxy. These stars immediately surround our solar system. Outside of this galaxy, there are trillions of stars that are sending energy to the trillions of cells in the human body. Relative to the plane of the Milky Way, our solar system is perpendicular, so that our North is facing the periphery of the galaxy.

The Milky Way contains billions of stars arranged in a huge spiral form. The stars in our galaxy correspond to our head and brain, while more distant or peripheral influences correspond with the cells of the body. The twelve constellations of astrology (for example, Taurus, Sagittarius, Libra, etc.) formed by distant galaxies combined with stars within our Milky Way, influence the body and form the twelve organ systems that are represented by the twelve meridians.

Between galaxies, there are invisible streams of energy that create galaxies when they intersect. These intergalactic currents are the same as the streams inside our body that are providing support for the cells. In other words, they are the blood, lymph, and body fluids.

Between our body and the galaxies that correspond an electromagnetic, or Ki charge is running. This can be seen as the electrical response between our cells changing from negative to positive to negative to positive. The spiral arms of the galaxy are receiving force centripetally and discharging it centrifugally. This spiral corresponds to the formation of the brain and nervous system. The brain is the center of the spiral of the nervous system and corresponds to the central disk of the Milky Way.

The thirty-two vertebrae of our spinal column correspond to the thirty-two stages of development that we can detect within the galaxy, as do the thirty-two teeth. If there were major sudden changes in the astronomical world (which would not happen easily), our body would change at that time in order to cope; if it did not, we could not live in the new environment. In an evolutionary sense, sudden galactic change is equal to mutation.

The cells at the outside of the skin correspond to nearby stars or galaxies, while the inside organs and tissues complement distant groups of stars. Specifically, the organs are formed at the inside as a result of distant galactic influence rather than individual influence of nearby stars. For this reason, organs are compact.

If you focus a camera at the North Star and leave the lens open for several hours, the exposed picture shows all the stars moving around one center, forming a spiral around the North Star. This is the spiral at the crown of our head. Again, set the camera at random and you will find many interesting patterns that correspond to our organs, glands, and chakras. From this general outline you can see that our body and the universe are corresponding and making balance.

To understand our body, we need to know the order of celestial movement, because each cell acts as a receiver and transmitter of heavenly influences. Most broadly this influence is manifested as motion of the constellations. If we view a composite map of the sky, the ecliptic is represented as a line running through the center of the map. This is apparent motion because in fact the earth is revolving around the sun.

The ecliptic corresponds to the diaphragm in the body and may be divided by twelve vertical lines the sun passes through each year. These twelve are the constellations of the zodiac. It is the movement of the constellations through the seasons that gives rise to the twelve meridians. Orion, which is located to the south of Taurus, is similar in form to the kidney; opposite this is Centaurus which is also the same size and shape as the kidney. Monoceros corresponds to the liver, and Canes Major, the gallbladder. Beneath Pices is Cetus, which corresponds to the stomach and spleen. Generally the territories above the line of the ecliptic correspond to the lungs, while the star groups beneath move in a spiral with the same pattern as the movement of the intestines. If you observe the night sky, you can see the vast concentration of our own galaxy, the Milky Way, which corresponds to the spine and nerves concentrated in the spinal cord.

In this way constellations or groups of constellations correspond to our organs, glands, and tissues. The twelve major constellations correspond to the twelve major meridians. Just as each organ has many cells, the stars that are visible to the naked eye are few compared with the billions within a galactic constellation. Each cell of the body is comprised of elements and individual atoms that are like the planets that orbit in distant solar systems. Furthermore, just as atoms have peripheral electrons, so planets have moons. In short, each of us is a universe; the stars in the heavens are our universal body, and our small self is within this universal body.

Celestial influences are changing each day; they appear and disappear and our body should follow this. If the influence of the stars is blocked in some way, a person will feel depressed and alone. When the influence is open he feels wonderful. Good health means that our organic body, which is a replica of the stars and constellations, is balancing and receiving full energy, or Ki from the surrounding universe.

Because the universe is expanding infinitely, our consciousness should be expanding infinitely also. For this our body should be more compact, not bloated or swollen. When we have an image of perfect stillness, it means we have no blockage. During the fall and winter, our thinking is clearest, although this is changing with the time of day or night. If you want to cultivate awareness of the infinite or the invisible spiritual world, meditate at two in the morning. For developing practical, down-to-earth consciousness, meditate at two in the afternoon.

Our body is nothing but a condensed form of the universe which has infinite depth. Beyond the stars which scientific instruments detect, there are others stretching infinitely into space. The same is true within our body; we can go infinitely in a microscopic direction. But the internal and external world are connected by food. If we do not balance food, necessarily we die. When we take in food it is a condensed form of the external universe; it is distributed throughout the body, and we make a new universe. This is complementary to our external body and makes balance with it.

The stars are the textbook by which we arrange ourselves and they are the order we imitate in daily life. If we become sick, it is because we have not followed the textbook properly. Finally, you can perceive our unique status; we are both the artist and the artist's creation. In other words, we have made ourselves and because we are free, we have the freedom to be healthy or sick.

All outer worlds are represented in the compact form of our body which is merely a finite representation of the universe. Our body has two aspects, internal and external, and this is really what is meant by man, but people are usually thinking only of the internal body. They do not think that the external body is their own, but both are ourselves. What then is the meaning of "I"? What is individual consciousness?

When the internal and external body are well balanced, our intuition works. Intuition is judgment based on the understanding of infinity. If this is unbalanced, we begin to have desire in order to restore balance. This desire takes the form of appetite for food or sex as well as intellectual curiosity or social harmony.

As a baby, we are still on the way toward coping with this expanded external universe, but we are not yet completely differentiated. In other words, our internal body is not completely formed and there is great desire. As we become adult, excessive desire should diminish and we go more and more by intuition. Unfortunately, modern people are eating chaotically, so that even though they become fully grown there is imbalance that causes excessive desire, frustration, and illness. Thus, people lose their health and stay at a lower level of consciousness.

Now you can begin to understand what you are and what it means to be human. When you see a galaxy in space, you are actually looking at yourself. The words "internal" and "external" are relative and interchangeable. You may reverse these, for what you are seeing is your own body. Our life is eternal although our body and cells are limited and always changing. You are always changing. You are infinity. If the heart is removed, you die, but if the sun or even some faraway galaxy is removed, you would die also. Far away and near, macrocosm and microcosm, both are your body, and there is no difference.

The Chakras in Healing

As we saw in Chapter 2, the chakras are found along the primary, or spiritual channel and control our physical, emotional, and mental functions. The first, or base chakra is the entrance for earth's force and exit for heaven's force. The seventh, or crown chakra is the entrance for heaven's force and exit for earth's force. The first chakra regulates the functions of the bladder and rectum, and also the reproductive organs. It controls part of the nervous and circulatory function. The first chakra, when working properly, creates physical and mental harmony with the environment and the ability to adapt to our surroundings. It also strengthens sexual vitality.

The second chakra is called *Tan-Den* in the Orient. It regulates digestion and absorption in the large and small intestines, and reproductive functions such as ovulation, pregnancy, childbirth, and the secretion of estrogen and progesterone. We call this area the *hara*, which means "ocean of Ki." The hara is the center of the body and is the seat of all physical vitality, including digestion, circulation, and reproduction. When this chakra is working properly, the hara generates physical stability and mental confidence.

The third chakra is in the region of the solar plexus. It deals with the digestive cycle, including the secretions of the stomach and the functions of the liver, gallbladder, pancreas, and spleen. It also influences the kidneys and adrenal glands. The fourth chakra is found in the heart region, and influences circulation and charges the blood and body fluids, including lymph, with Ki. In the Orient, the heart chakra is called *Dan-Chu*. The heart chakra also influences digestive and respiratory functions, and in general, controls our emotions.

Chakra number five is found in the throat area. It controls the functions of respiration and speech. It influences the motion of the tongue and charges the saliva and the mouth with Ki. The throat chakra also regulates expression. The sixth chakra is in the area of the midbrain, and controls our consciousness and physical reactions. It deals primarily with intuition, while the second chakra, the hara, deals with instinct. The seventh chakra is located in the area of the hair spiral on top of the head. It controls the unified functions of our spiritual, mental, and physical activities. When this chakra is active, we develop universal understanding.

The chakras are, of course, interrelated, so their functions are not exclusive. They interact with one another and influence all of the body's functions to one degree or another. The fourth chakra, the heart, influences not only the heart and circulation, but also the lungs. The third chakra influences not only the stomach but all the other organs in the center of the body, such as the liver, kidneys, and spleen.

The heart chakra is positioned between the midbrain, which is the central chakra of the head, and the hara, which is the central chakra of the body. The hara is the center of the digestive system. It creates confidence and security. It has a stabilizing effect on our Ki flow as a whole. The heart chakra deals with emotion, sentiment, and security. It is the center of the circulatory system. The midbrain deals with thinking and consciousness, and is the center of the nervous system.

Meditation causes the spiritual channel and chakras to become open, active, and receptive to heaven and earth. That is actually the main purpose of meditation and other forms of spiritual practice. Meditation, breath control, and chanting make the chakras and spiritual channel active and clear. When we chant certain sounds or practice specific breathing techniques, we emphasize certain chakras and from there different physical, mental, and spiritual results are produced.

These and other spiritual practices are actually part of holistic healing. Holistic healing has two areas: one is to bring abnormal conditions back to normal and the other is to provide everyone with the basis for health and a deeper awareness of life. In the first category of healing, we use diet, simple home care, and energy treatments such as palm healing and massage. There are many applications in the second category, including exercise, ethics or morality, religion, spiritual practices, and others. These practices and teachings have various names, but in general, they are all part of the medicine of humanity. Doctors of the first category need to know how to use balanced diet, special foods and drinks, external applications such as ginger compress, and energy treatments such as palm healing and massage to correct energy imbalances and restore health. In addition to being able to use these simple natural methods to help people recover from sickness, doctors in the second category are able to help people develop their fullest potential. Doctors in this category are not only physical and mental advisers, but philosophers, educators, and guides for the way of life, including physical, mental, and spiritual issues. This type of doctor can help families, communities, and society, and is able to establish world peace.

The Spiritual Cause of Sickness

If the chakras are not working properly, or if the spiritual channel is not functioning well, a variety of problems appear throughout the body. The spiritual channel is the main channel of life energy. If the chakras or spiritual channel become hard or rigid, blocked by deposits of fat and mucus, or loose from the intake of sugar, drugs, or alcohol, then life energy will not flow properly. All sickness is caused, more or less, by problems with the spiritual channel and chakras.

Multiple sclerosis (MS) offers a clear example. When I came to the United States more than forty years ago, I was not aware that this disease existed, but now I am seeing more and more people who have it. In this disease the legs do not work; gradually the arms do not work, and the ability to speak may also diminish. According to modern medicine, there is no cure for multiple sclerosis. However, an understanding of the chakras can help us see the cause of multiple sclerosis. Ki or energy is continuously flowing from the hara to the legs, charging and vitalizing them. But in MS, Ki does not run smoothly to the legs. The overall charge of energy becomes weak, and so do the legs. Ki also flows along the meridians to the arms, but if it becomes weak, the arms eventually become paralyzed. In the same way, if the throat chakra is not working well, if the charge of Ki is not running smoothly, the tongue cannot move, the thyroid and parathyroid glands do not work well, and the person cannot speak.

Dysfunction in the chakras also affects the endocrine system. Blockage of chakra energy can disrupt the secretion of pituitary, pancreatic, adrenal, and sexual hormones. All disorders of the endocrine system are related to the condition of the spiritual channel and chakras.

Tests of Flexibility

We can see whether the primary channel and chakras are charging well by checking our overall degree of flexibility. If the charge of Ki is going smoothly, then all of our functions and activities are smooth and efficient, including our physical and mental activities. When the telephone rings, if you immediately pick it up and say, "Hello. How are you? Can I help you?" your energy is flowing actively. But if you are slow or lazy, that means your chakras and spiritual channel are not charging actively.

Characteristics such as adaptability, accuracy, and speediness are signs that the spiritual channel and chakras are functioning properly. On the other hand, rigidity, stubbornness, arrogance, slowness, and laziness are signs that the spiritual channel and chakras are not working well. If they are not working at all, this is the state we call *death*. Death means there is no electromagnetic charge running through the body, so our systems do not function anymore. No longer can we hear, see, feel, or react. To be alive means that the chakras, spiritual channel, meridians, and meridian branches are actively charged with energy. The distinction between life and death is therefore determined by whether or not energy is charging the body. To the extent that energy is flowing actively and smoothly, we are healthy and alive.

There are many ways to check the condition of the chakras and spiritual channel and how well Ki is flowing through them. Below are several methods:

1. Since Ki is flowing from the chakras to the arms and hands, seeing whether the arms, hands, and fingers are flexible or not tells us how well Ki is flowing. To test this, bend your arms and put your palms together in front of you in the prayer position, attaching the fingers. Now try to bend the wrists and palms to a ninety-degree angle so that the palms are parallel to the floor. If you are able to do this, the Ki flow in this area is going well. If you cannot, your body has become rigid and your energy flow stagnant.

2. To test how well energy is flowing in the lower body, especially in the hara, have the person you wish to check lie on their back. Ask them to bend the knees and put both feet flat on the floor a few inches from the hips. Ask them to put the knees together, and to breathe slowly and relax. To check for hardness, pain, or tightness in the intestinal region, push in, gently but deeply, along the intestine as the person slowly exhales. When you feel hardness or if there is pain, it is a sign that the flow of energy in the lower body is blocked.

3. Another way to test for flexibility is to move your right arm across the front of your face, along the left side of the head, across the back of the head and try to grasp or at least touch your right ear. Many people cannot do this, and this rigidity is reflected in their thinking and behavior.

4. Another way to check for overall flexibility is to lay down on your stomach. Bend your knees and try to touch your buttocks with your heels. Then try to attach your heels to the floor on either side of your hips. Use your hands to pull your legs down.

When energy is flowing actively, it effects every aspect of life. Our personality and behavior, for example, are reflections of how well energy is flowing. (The Japanese word for personality, *Ki-Sho*, means "Ki nature" or "Ki character.") All of these ways, and there are many more, are showing whether or not heaven's and earth's forces are charging well throughout our body. If the charge of Ki is going smoothly, then naturally our brain is active and alert, our heart is functioning naturally, and our speaking, breathing, digestion, and sexual functions are coordinating with each other and proceeding actively.

Problems arise when Ki flow is impaired because of rigidity, fatty accumulation, or looseness throughout the body. If your body is rigid, you cannot react immediately and instinctively to changes in your environment or daily life. When cold weather comes, or when heat or strong winds come, then you cannot adapt. If some difficulty comes in your life—if you lose your job, money, or separate from your husband or wife—you cannot cope successfully. Or if war or other social difficulties arise, you cannot cope, and cannot tolerate new situations because of tightness or rigidity in body and mind. So you can act only in a certain way. And when circumstances change, you have difficulty responding appropriately or turning difficulties into opportunities.

A Centered Diet

In order for our Ki flow to be charged to the maximum, and to flow smoothly and clearly through the spiritual channel and chakras, it is necessary to eat well. Eating well means eating a balanced natural diet in harmony with the environment and personal needs. The principle of yin and yang is invaluable in helping us understand the type of energy foods contain and in creating dynamic balance in our diets.

Among foods there are yin and yang types. Some foods have stronger expansive energy, others have stronger contracting energy. Cereal grains are generally balanced, although, as we will see, certain varieties are more yang and others more yin. Beans are more yin than grains—they are larger and higher in fat, and that is why it is better to eat them in small quantities. Eating too many beans can cause Ki flow to stagnate and thinking to become dull.

Vegetables are more yin than grains or beans. Cooked vegetables are more yang than raw vegetables, and temperate varieties are more yang than tropical varieties. The roots of vegetables are more yang and the leaves more yin. Vegetables that grow in the summer are yin in comparison to those that grow in fall or winter. Fruits, especially tropical varieties, are yin in comparison to vegetables, and sugar, drugs, and medications are far more expansive and yin than fruits.

Oil is strongly yin, so when you sauté or fry foods, it is better to use only a small amount. Oil is a partial food. It is extracted from grains and seeds. It was traditionally used for the purpose of cooking. Oil is yin, so it attracts fire, which is yang. Oil makes food cook quickly. But the oils and fats that our bodies need for nourishment are best taken as a part of whole foods. Whole grains and beans contain natural oils and fats. It is better to take these substances as a part of the foods themselves, rather than in an extracted form.

As we go in the opposite direction—toward yang—we find animal foods: fish, then poultry, meat, and eggs. Among the varieties of cheese, some are more yang, others more yin. Goat cheese and other hard, salty cheeses are yang. Soft, less salty cheeses are yin. Milk, yogurt, and ice cream are also yin.

There are also yin and yang varieties of grains. Buckwheat is the most yang grain, while corn, which ripens in the summer, is the most yin. Brown rice is generally balanced. It ripens in the fall, during a time when the weather is not too cold and not too warm. Wheat is also balanced, but a little more yin than rice. Generally our eating should go toward the center. However, between yin and yang, which one should we depend on more, in terms of volume? We need to take a larger volume of yin, meaning that in normal circumstances, we should base our diet on plants, rather than on animal foods.

The ratio between heaven's downward force and earth's upward force at the surface of the planet is about seven to one. That means heaven's force is roughly seven times stronger than earth's force. In order to balance our planetary environment, therefore, we need to eat the inverse of this ratio, or in other words, seven times more yin than yang in our diets.

The use of fire in cooking, makes food yang. It brings the energy of grains, beans, vegetables, and other plant foods closer to the center. When we use strong yin foods, we need stronger cooking (more fire) to bring them to a balanced point. When we use strong yang foods, then lighter cooking is better. For example, the Eskimo live in a very cold region, and must use animal food to balance their environment. But they usually do not cook this animal food, or cook it lightly. In a similar way, when people in the Orient eat eggs on occasion, they do not cook them. They mix the egg with a little tamari soy sauce and eat it raw. Fish is also eaten raw in Oriental countries. In Japanese, raw fish is known as sashimi. Eating animal food in this way produces less extreme effects, as does eating it in small amounts with plenty of vegetables.

From a biological standpoint, it is better to avoid meat unless you live in a far-northern climate. Mammals are our next of kin, and it is better not to eat them. They are too close to us on the evolutionary scale and are high in cholesterol and saturated fat. Poultry is also not recommended for regular consumption in temperate climates. The quality of modern poultry is so poor that it is best avoided. Chickens today are fed artificial growth hormones and antibiotics, and are frequently infected with salmonella and other bacteria. Moreover, poultry is now being irradiated in the United States. Even with these problems, however, many people believe that chicken is a healthy food, and it has recently replaced red meat as the most commonly consumed animal food in the United States. In a temperate climate, the safest form of animal food is low-fat, white-meat fish. It can be eaten once or twice a week if desired, along with the main meal of whole grains and vegetables.

Men and women have different dietary needs, especially in regard to the intake of animal food. A woman's nature is enhanced by earth's expanding energy. If she eats more toward yin, and especially less animal food, her condition becomes harmonious with her inner nature. Many women know this intuitively, and are less attracted to animal food than men. But modern eating habits are based on the regular consumption of animal food.

The modern diet is making many women become overly masculine. Many women experience hormone imbalances and menstrual disorders, and develop facial and body hair, as a result of eating too much animal food.

After eating strong yang food, people are attracted to the opposite extreme, including foods such as sugar, tropical fruit, chocolate, and soft drinks. By this they try to make balance with the strong yang energy of animal foods. Men can generally afford to eat a little more animal food than women, provided the overall ratio of animal to plant food does not exceed about one to seven. But today men are eating foods such as steak, hamburger, eggs, and chicken every day, and in some cases, at every meal. They become excessively masculine, and must eventually counter this by eating sugar, tropical fruit, ice cream, and other extremely yin foods. As a result, they start to lose male energy.

Some men eat excessively yin foods alone, without eating eggs, chicken, and meat. As a result, they develop female characteristics. An increasing number of men are developing breasts, and there are about 4,000 cases of male breast cancer in the United States each year. The growth hormones fed to cattle, chickens, and other livestock, all of which are extremely yin, contributes to these conditions.

Modern eating habits are also the cause of attraction to vegetarian, fruitarian, lacto-vegetarian, raw foods, and raw fruit diets. In many cases, people who have eaten plenty of animal food in the past eventually exceed their constitutional tolerance for yang, and start to consume a more yin diet. (Alcohol abuse, for example, is usually caused by a past history of too much animal food.) A person in this condition may temporarily become better, more balanced, but since these forms of yin are very strong, eventually they erase their history of extreme yang. If they continue to take extremely yin foods and drinks, an overly yin condition arises. Then the intestines become loose, skin troubles begin, and thinking becomes dull and obscure. A variety of physical and mental problems stem from this condition. A person in this condition must eventually come back to the middle if they wish to establish good health.

Macrobiotic eating is not balancing by extremes. It is based on centered foods. Through the use of fire in cooking, we make each meal balanced with the environment and our daily life. Macrobiotics is not a rigid diet. It changes according to each person's condition and environment. Someone may eat 50 percent grain, another person may eat grain as 80 percent of the meal, someone may eat fish once or twice a week, someone else may not eat it at all. Some people may eat raw vegetables, while someone else may not. Minor adjustments such as these need to be made on an individual basis.

When a person eats a very yang diet, for example, plenty of meat, cheese, chicken, and eggs, the primary channel and chakras become hard and rigid as fat and cholesterol accumulate in and around the organs. If we eat a very yin diet, the chakras become loose and open. In order to recover a balanced condition, we need to eat centrally balanced foods, using whole grains as primary foods, with side dishes of vegetables, sea vegetables, and beans, plus occasional supplementary foods such as white-meat fish and seasonal fruit. Through cooking, we bring these foods closer to central balance. By this balanced way of eating, your condition will gradually become cleaner and the flow of Ki will run smoothly through your body.

Artificial Interference in the Body

Many conditions are accelerated, along with chaotic eating habits, by artificial interference with life, such as operations to remove organs and parts of the body. Let us take a simple example.

The intestines are hollow and long, or more yin. Their natural tendency is to become loose and expanded. Even though they are compressed into a small space, and squeezed like an accordion, moving in and out from both sides, the intestines are yin in terms of size and structure. In order to function properly, however, the intestinal tract needs yang energy to make balance, otherwise it would have no contracting power and could not absorb or move food along. What is the yang organ in this area? The appendix is small, compact, and yang. It makes balance with the expanded structure of the small and large intestines.

As biological evolution progressed, the intestines became longer. At one time, the appendix was larger. But gradually, as the intestines became more expanded, the appendix became contracted as a counterpoint. Many doctors think that because the appendix is small and inactive, it does not have a function, so whenever there is a problem, they remove it.

However, when the appendix is suddenly removed, there is only yin in this area, so the intestines become loose. Indigestion, constipation, diarrhea, and weakening of the legs may start. Unless the person eats well, he may suffer from digestive disorders. If you have not had your appendix removed, then even though you binge occasionally, you do not create much indigestion, diarrhea, or other symptoms. But if you have had your appendix removed, even a modest amount of binging can create problems.

In the female body, the hara is where conception takes place, where the placenta is formed and where the embryo grows. There is a great concentration of energy in this area during pregnancy. When pregnancy arises, heaven's and earth's forces charge this area intensively, blood starts to gather here, and intense activity begins. During pregnancy, a woman's body is becoming yang; there is greater activity in the hara chakra, along with a concentration of energy and blood. Today, however, many women have an operation to remove the fetus and stop the pregnancy, causing these energies to suddenly disperse. Strong yang suddenly changes into yin, causing the entire lower body to become weaker.

The same thing happens when we pick the fruit from a tree before it ripens. As the fruit starts to mature, a great deal of energy is concentrated toward it. If we pick that fruit, the entire tree is influenced. The roots, stem, leaves, and tree as a whole become weak. The same thing happens after an abortion. The hara becomes weaker, as does the body as a whole. Then chronic problems begin in the intestines, the legs become weaker, and the woman's overall health declines.

By eating macrobiotically, a woman can recover from these effects. General physical recovery can be achieved in about six months, depending on the woman's overall state of health. But many women do not know how to eat well, and after having an abortion continue eating tropical fruits, sugar, nightshade vegetables, and soft drinks, or continue using drugs, alcohol, or medications. Then the hara region, intestines, and body as a whole cannot be repaired smoothly. These items interfere with the process of recovery.

Treating the Chakras

These and other artificial procedures cause the chakras and primary channel to become dull, weak, and inactive. As a result, people are loosing flexibility, adaptability, and vitality. Artificial procedures also cause our thinking power, consciousness, and spirituality to become weaker. Restoring the chakras to a normal condition, in which energy is charging fully, is the central issue in healing. The macrobiotic approach to multiple sclerosis (MS) is an example of one method of chakra healing. Of course, in order to recover completely, a person with MS needs to avoid extremes and base their diet on centrally balanced foods. However, it is possible to charge the chakras from the outside in order to help the person recover full energy more quickly.

If a person with MS eats well and keeps active, he can still recover without receiving external treatments. But many people with MS are confined to a wheelchair and are not active. It therefore takes longer for them to recover with diet alone. The healing process can be accelerated by charging the chakras from the outside. Instead of approaching the chakras from the front, which in this case would be too strong, we can approach them from the back, which is a gentle way of charging the body with energy.

Traditional healers used a technique known as moxibustion for this purpose. Moxa is made of dried mugwort leaves. A piece of moxa is rolled into a small ball, about the size of a grain of rice, and put on an acupuncture point. It is then lit with a stick of incense. The moxa burns and at the last moment, energy charges the point, at which time, the person feels heat. Vibrations go toward the inside of the body or along the meridians, and strong energy charges the organs and chakras. Acupuncture is based on the same principle. In acupuncture, metal needles are inserted in the points in order to conduct energy from the atmosphere, in the way that a television antenna picks up signals. Acupuncture and moxibustion are both effective, yet both have drawbacks.

If a person is depending on acupuncture, then every several days he must go to the clinic, while if moxa is used directly on the skin, it leaves a small black mark. The mark usually disappears in several weeks if the procedure is repeated only once or twice. But to help someone recover from MS, treatments need to be given repeatedly over several months, or until the patient is hopefully able to stand up and walk. However, if a mark is left on the skin every time moxa is applied, the skin could eventually rupture. Instead of applying moxa directly to the skin, a less direct method can be used. Traditional healers used sticks of moxa for this purpose. Moxa sticks look like cigars that are packed with dried mugwort. An ordinary cigarette can be substituted if moxa sticks are not available.

When MS reaches an advanced stage, the spine shows signs of sclerosis, or in other words, calcification and hardening. As a result, the nerves do not work well. Hardening or rigidity along the spine, which many people have, is actually the beginning of MS. Even mild sclerosis interferes with the transmission of nervous impulses and blocks the flow of Ki through the chakras. It is possible to detect sclerosis by having someone lie on their stomach, completely relaxed, and pressing gently along the spine with the thumbs. If you detect hardness in any part of the spine, it is a sign that sclerosis is beginning.

The condition of the heart, hara, and stomach chakras is especially important in MS. Hardening develops in and around these chakras, blocking nerve impulses to the arms and legs. At the same time, these chakras can be used to activate the nervous system and flow of chakra and meridian energy to the arms and legs. To treat these chakras, have the person lie on his stomach and use your thumbs to push gently between the vertebrae in the upper spine in the area corresponding to the heart chakra. A person with MS will usually feel some pain when you push. Place a mark wherever the person feels pain, and then do the same with the region of the spine corresponding to the stomach and hara chakras. A person with MS will normally feel pain or sensitivity whenever you press behind the middle and lower chakras, as will people with weakness in the legs from having had an abortion or their appendix removed.

If you are treating the person with stick or cigarette moxa, approach the painful points with the lit end of the stick. Ask the person to tell you when the point feels hot. Approach and slowly circle the point until the patient feels hot, then move away. Approach again and then pull away. Do this five to ten times before moving on to the next point. Treat the points one by one. If you are treating a person who cannot move his arms or legs, his limbs may start to jerk while you are giving the treatment. That is evidence that energy is shooting along the meridians and activating the nerves. Even a healthy person will experience a feeling of lightness or tingling in the arms and legs following treatment.

Moxa is a strong form of treatment, so it is not necessary to repeat it every day. It can be done once every three days in the beginning, and when the patient starts to walk, every five or seven days. Of course the patient must eat well, otherwise even though the chakras are being stimulated externally, the underlying cause will not have been changed.

This simple but effective treatment takes about ten minutes. The patient's family can learn how to do it. If the patient's progress seems slow, simple adjustments in the treatment may be necessary. For example, you may need to treat different places on the back, or treat each point longer. You may also need to bring the moxa closer to the point, so that the person feels definite heat, rather than just a mild feeling of warmth. The treatment must be strong enough to produce a sensation of heat in order for healing to occur. It is therefore important to continually monitor the results of the treatment and adjust the method when necessary. To check the condition of the primary channel and chakras in general, have the person lie on his back. Ask him to bend his legs and put his feet on the floor near the hips so that the knees are sticking up in the air. He can relax and breathe in and out slowly. Then, as he breathes out, push deeply but gently along the intestines to check for hardness and pain. Many people have hardness here and naturally feel pain when you apply pressure. Press along the large intestine and then in the region of the small intestine. This simple method reveals the overall condition of the primary channel and chakras, especially how well Ki is flowing through these pathways.

Drug-Free Headache Relief

The same principles can be used to bring drug-free relief from headaches. Headaches represent an energy imbalance and, depending on the type of energy involved, appear in different regions of the head. Some headaches appear in the front of the head, others appear on the sides, and others at the back of the head. Headaches also develop deep inside the head. Each of type of headache has a different cause.

The front part of the head is bigger, more expanded, while the back is tight and compact. The front is yin, and the back is yang. Strong yin produces greater disharmony in the front of the head, while strong yang creates disharmony in the back. The sides of the head are expanded, but less so than the front. Pain in the front of the head is caused by strong yin and pain on either side is caused by mild yin. The back of the head is yang, but the deep inside regions are very yang. Headaches in the back of the head are caused by strong yang; those deep inside by very strong yang. We now have four causes of headaches: strong yin and mild yin and very strong yang and moderately strong yang.

If someone eats sugar or fruit juice, or takes birth control pills, aspirin, or other medications or extreme yin foods, the front part of the head will be affected more. When eaten in excess, lesser yin foods affect the sides. If you eat fish or salty foods, pain appears in the back of the head. If you eat very strong yang, then the center, deep inside, becomes troubled. Eggs, smoked salmon, bacon, liver, caviar, and ginseng are examples of very strong yang.

Headaches in the front of the head are caused by too much fruit, soft drinks, sugar, honey, chocolate and medication, vitamin C, birth control pills, and other yin extremes. Headaches on the sides are caused by oily, greasy foods, including ketchup, potato chips, or too much fresh or dried fruit. Herbal teas, including stimulant, aromatic teas like peppermint and chamomile, also contribute to side headaches.

Alcohol can also produce headaches. Wine affects the front of the head, while beer tends to affect the sides. Wine is made from fruit and is more yin; beer is made from grain and is more yang. Strong alcohol is very yin and when taken in excess, tends to produce pain in the front of the head.

Yin foods produce expansion. Fruit juice makes the brain cells expand and so do aspirin, alcohol, chocolate, and antibiotics. In order to make these cells contract, we need to apply cold. Cold towels can be used to help bring relief from headaches in the front and sides of the head. Headaches in the back of the head are caused by too much contracting energy. Hot towels cause the cells to expand and thus can be used for this type of headache. We cannot reach the deep inner regions of the head directly, but we can treat the back of the neck, and by that stimulate deep inside the head. Placing a hot towel around the neck helps the person relax and eases deep tension headaches.

Using the Meridians

Adjusting the flow of energy along the meridians can help relieve headaches. The head is opposite and complementary to the feet and toes. Certain meridians extend from the head down to the toes. The section of the meridian that runs along the head is complementary to the section that runs through the toes. By stimulating one part, we produce an effect in the opposite part.

The stomach meridian runs across the front of the head. It also runs through the second and third toes. Massaging the second and third toes can help bring relief from headaches in the front of the head. The bladder meridian runs across the top of the head and down the back of the neck. For headaches in the back part of the head, we can massage the bladder meridian on the fifth toe. The gallbladder meridian comes to the sides of the head. It is a complicated meridian. Headaches in this part of the head can be relieved by massaging the fourth toe. Deep tension headaches can be relieved by stimulating the spleen and liver meridians that run through the first toe. Now let us see how to apply this understanding practically.

Suppose someone comes down with a headache in the front of the head. We know from the location that her headache is caused by too much strong yin. So to help her we need to apply cold to the front of her head and treat the second and third toes. To do this, ask her to lie down comfortably on her back. Run a cotton towel under the cold faucet, wring it out, and place it on her forehead. Then go around to her feet, grasp the toes of both feet by placing them between your thumbs and index fingers, pull outward to the extent that her whole body moves slightly, and then relax. You may do the second toe first, and then the third, or you may do both at the same time. Repeat this procedure for about five minutes.

If her headache is centered on the sides of the head, then massage the fourth toe. You may also apply cold towels to the forehead. If the headache is toward the back, have her lie down on her stomach. Then pull and massage the bladder meridian on the fifth toe as described above. Place a hot towel on the back of her neck. If the headache is deep inside, ask her to lie on her back then pull and massage the first toe while placing a hot towel around the neck.

Energy Balance in the Organs

All of the organs contribute in some way to the overall balance of energy in the body. The liver and spleen, for example, maintain a vital balance between the energies of heaven and earth. The liver is charged primarily by the flow of earth's ascending force which is stronger on the right side of the body, and the spleen by the downward flow of heaven's force which is stronger on the left. If the balance between the liver and spleen is disturbed, we cannot maintain an upright posture. The balance between left and right also regulates the body's energy level as a whole. The complementary/antagonistic energies of the liver and pancreas (located on the left side of the body) regulate the level of sugar in the blood. When this balance is disturbed, we develop either diabetes or hypoglycemia. The kidneys maintain a similar balance, although in a subtle way. The kidneys regulate the volume of minerals and liquids in the body, and contribute to our upright form and posture.

The balance between other organs contributes to our erect posture. The heart and small intestine, and the lungs and large intestine balance the strong yin energy existing in the upper body and the strong yang energy in the lower body.

All postural problems belong to one of these four basic types; in other words, there is some problem with one of these four dimensions of balance. Within these four, two—the heart and small intestine and liver and spleen—are extremely vital, to the extent that if either one becomes seriously troubled, our vertical form will collapse. Maintaining a vertical posture depends on the balance between these organs. We can refer to the horizontal balance between the liver and spleen, and vertical balance between the heart and small intestine as the "cross balance" of the body.

If there is major problem in the heart, like a heart attack, or if someone is kicked or hit in the small intestine—he cannot maintain this cross balance, and must collapse. Or, if the liver suddenly becomes unbalanced, a person also loses vital balance and collapses. A good example of this is epilepsy.

Origin and Treatment of Epilepsy

According to modern medicine, epilepsy is an incurable disease. However, the mechanism of epilepsy is actually quite simple. With time and patience, a person with this disease can recover. There is no medication that can actually cure epilepsy, but through the macrobiotic diet and way of life, recovery can be achieved.

In the brain, bundles of nerve fibers are interspersed among the brain cells. When brain cells become very expanded, they press against the nerve fibers; naturally, the cells cannot function in a normal way and begin to send strong, desperate signals. If this happens in the conscious part of the brain, then hallucinations or delirium arise. But when this happens toward the rear of the brain, where reflexes and unconscious functions are centered, the result is a seizure.

What makes brain cells expand? In the case of hallucinations, the cause is usually strong yin, including drugs, sugar, or medication. However, when overexpansion arises in the yang, rear portion of the brain, the underlying cause stems from the overintake of milder forms of yin over a long period of time. When this condition suddenly becomes acute, a seizure arises. Epilepsy is commonly caused by too much liquid, fruit, alcohol, raw vegetables, tomatoes and other nightshades, in combination with the intake of stronger yin such as medication, sugar, and ice cream. The steady intake of these foods depletes the minerals in the body. Eventually, there are not enough minerals in the blood to maintain a sufficient degree of contraction in the cells. Over time, the depletion of minerals causes the cells in the brain to gradually expand.

Epileptic seizures frequently occur on rainy days, when the volume of liquid in the body easily becomes excessive; or early in the morning, when earth's rising energy in the atmosphere is stronger. They are common after a person with this chronic condition drinks alcohol, or after holidays when people tend to eat a larger than normal amount of sugar, fruit, or sweets. The intake of strong yin causes their condition to suddenly become acute.

Once we understand the energy imbalances underlying these conditions, we can develop simple methods of treatment aimed at restoring balance. For example, the liver is related to the back part of the brain. The visual center is located here, and thus the liver and eyes are related. The spleen and pancreas are also related to the eyes. During an epileptic seizure, earth's expanding energy becomes much too excessive, activating the liver. At the same time, the spleen, which is charged by heaven's downward force on the left side of the body, becomes severely inhibited.

The movement of energy during a seizure follows the Ko cycle of the five transformations described in Chapter 1. The liver corresponds to upward, or tree energy, while the spleen represents downward, soil energy. Tree and soil energy are opposite and complementary. When tree energy becomes active, it produces a suppressing or inhibiting effect on soil energy. Moreover, in Oriental medicine, the liver corresponds to the spiritual function of "soul," while the spleen represents the intellect. During a seizure, the intellect is totally suppressed, and the soul becomes wild and overactive. At the same time, the liver meridian becomes so overcharged that it releases energy in a violent spasm. Traditional holistic treatments for epileptic seizures were aimed at restoring balance to the liver and spleen meridians.

The energy treatment for epilepsy makes use of points located at the end of the liver and spleen meridians. These points, known as *Sei points*, are located in the part of the body that is opposite to the head. The Sei points for the liver and spleen are on the large toe, on either side of the base of the nail. These points appear at the periphery of the meridian, and correspond to the innermost regions of the organ.

When someone is struck with a seizure, it may be necessary to place a stick in the person's mouth, in order to prevent him from biting or swallowing his tongue. A bamboo chopstick is good for this purpose. Then, using the thumbs, apply strong pressure to the nail of the large toe, treating both toes at the same time, while also pulling the toes outward in order to draw excess energy down away from the head. This can be done in a rhythmic fashion—pressing and releasing, pressing and releasing—

until the person comes out of the seizure. This simple energy treatment can help someone having a seizure regain consciousness after a minute or two. Placing a cold towel on the back of the head causes brain cells to contract, and can also be helpful. Of course, in order for a person to recover from epilepsy, it is necessary to change the underlying cause by changing the way the person eats and drinks. A balanced macrobiotic diet, modified slightly to emphasize yang factors, is necessary to achieve a lasting remission.

The principles of energy balancing can be applied in the emergency treatment for heart attack. The Sei points for the heart and small intestine are located at the tip of the little finger on both hands. The heartbeat can be stabilized or strengthened by grasping the tips of both little fingers between the thumb and index finger and pressing hard and releasing, pressing and releasing, in a steady rhythm for several minutes. As we can see, the understanding of energy, including knowledge of the meridians and points, can help us discover many simple, effective, and uncomplicated treatments.

Correcting Energy Imbalances

Traditional philosopher-healers did not limit their view of the human body to its chemical or physical substances only. Their view of human life, human sickness, and human medicine was oriented by their understanding of energy. They considered all conditions as belonging to either of two categories: those resulting from underactive or deficient energy, and those resulting from overactive or excessive energy. Later the ancient Chinese called these categories *Kyo*, literally "empty symptom," or lack of energy, and *Jitsu*, literally "full symptoms," or excessive energy.

For example, if someone becomes malnourished, or if their heart becomes weak and blood pressure drops, this would be considered Kyo. If someone has a high fever, frequent coughing or sweating, or if someone is overweight, their condition would be classified as Jitsu.

Traditional healers also classified medicines into two categories: those that supply energy and thus activate the body; and those that draw excessive energy out of the body and thus calm it down. They would select certain foods, herbs, special plants, or in some cases minerals or animal foods, and use them for their energy properties.

The way of selecting and choosing the right treatment went according to either of several principles. For example, suppose someone develops a high fever; that means excessive energy (Jitsu) is trying to discharge. In order to relieve that fever, there are two basic ways: (1) we can use a calming medicine, to reduce that overactivity and make those rough vibrations cease; in this case, a good example would be kuzu drink with a little umeboshi and tamari soy sauce; (2) the other way would be to accelerate that vibration by activating it strongly, giving something like grated daikon or boiled orange peel; in that case, the fever's energy would become active and quickly burn away in the form of sweating.

The first approach is more harmonious, and would be safer to use for a person whose health is delicate; the second approach is more drastic, but may work very rapidly, and is usually easier to use for a person who is stronger. A modern version of this second method is aspirin; that is the same basic approach as taking raw daikon for a fever. Only aspirin is more powerful and creates additional problems. Using their understanding of Kyo and Jitsu, traditional healers were able to create many effective treatments without dangerous side effects.

Calming and Activating Treatments

The principle of energy balancing applies not only to food and herbal medicine, but to other holistic therapies, such as shiatsu, acupuncture, and external applications such as ginger compresses. All of these healing techniques can be classified as either energy-activating or energy-calming. Acupuncture, for example, can actually work either way, depending on the specific technique: if a needle is left in for some time, it gradually begins to send energy deep inside the body, activating the meridian and organ. But if the needle is inserted for a short time only, and withdrawn with a gentle clockwise motion, the effect is to draw energy out of the body. Moxibustion is an energy-supplying, activating treatment. It can be helpful for conditions such as constipation or weak, tired kidneys. However, it is not helpful in cases of inflammation or fever. In these instances, energy is already overactive and applying additional heat to the body can make them worse.

What kind of effect does a ginger compress (towels dipped in hot ginger water and applied to the body) have? This is generally an energy-activating or energy-supplying treatment; the corresponding energy-diminishing treatment would be a cold compress, such as a chlorophyll, tofu, or ice plaster. As examples, if a person's intestines are sluggish and not absorbing well, you can apply a ginger compress to activate that function. On the other hand, it would be dangerous to give a ginger compress to someone with appendicitis or pneumonia, both of which are symptoms of excessive, overactive energy; in those cases, a cold treatment helps draw out energy and reduce the overactivity of those conditions. In the case of cancer, which is again a symptom of excessive energy building up in the form of active cancer cells, we are careful not to apply ginger compress for more than a few minutes, or just long enough to stimulate the flow of blood to and from that area; and then we follow that with a cold, energy-reducing or drawing-out treatment, usually a taro plaster.

Again, like acupuncture, if you have good understanding, you can adapt shiatsu techniques to have either type of effect, either strongly supplying energy to certain parts of the body, or calmly drawing excessive energy out of the body. People who are just beginning to practice shiatsu may have overactive energy when they treat, particularly if they are eating too much animal food, liquid, sweets, or even simply eating too much in general; and it may be difficult to practice an energy-calming type of shiatsu. But a skilled practitioner is able to freely adjust his or her technique to suit any type of condition.

Palm Healing

Palm healing is an important holistic practice. In palm healing, we use the energy generated in the hands, which we receive from heaven and earth, to directly accelerate a person's energy and self-healing abilities. The right hand is charged with earth's yin, centrifugal force, while the left is charged with heaven's yang, centripetal force. The left hand has the effect of supplying energy, or further activating energy; this is appropriate to use in the case of a symptom that is Kyo, or deficient. The right hand calms or draws out energy, and is appropriate when the person's symptom is Jitsu or overactive.

Today, most health problems are caused by stagnation from overeating in general or from an excess of certain types of foods; so when you practice palm healing, it is more practical to use your right hand, to dissolve and draw out stagnation. In other words, most conditions are best relieved by encouraging the elimination of excessive or stagnated energy; a fever is a good example of this. But in some cases, you may need to use your left hand more, when there is some deficient, weak symptom.

You can also vary this effect by using different parts of your hand. We can divide the hand into three areas: (1) the peripheral area, or fingertips; energy from the meridians gathers there, giving off and picking up energy from the atmosphere; (2) the intermediate area, or roots of the fingers; and (3) the central area, the center of the palm itself. If you want to supply energy, the central region, the palm itself can be used. The center of the palm is the most actively charged region of the hand. If you want to draw energy out, lightly apply the fingertips. For an intermediate effect, apply the roots of the fingers, or even the hand as a whole.

Practical Guidelines For Palm Healing

There are several important points to keep in mind for good palm healing. For your body to be charging well, keep your spine straight; then if you hold your hands out in front of your body, and hold the intention or image of sending energy strongly in your mind, normally this energy projects for a distance of about three or four meters (although with the right image in your mind, you can actually project this energy for hundreds of miles.) If your attention and image falter, this power is greatly diminished; so when you are palm healing, hold in mind the image that you are an empty vessel, receiving and projecting heaven's and earth's forces to cleanse and heal that person.

When you place your palm on the person, it is better to apply no pressure, or only light pressure. Pushing down hard increases physical contact, and decreases the effectiveness of the vibrational contact you are using. Also, do not allow any other part of your body to touch the person; this in effect short-circuits the energy you are sending or withdrawing, reducing the effectiveness of the treatment. A light covering of clothing, ideally cotton, is actually preferable to direct contact with the skin; if at all possible, synthetic clothing should be avoided, for both you and the other person.

While you are applying your hands, hold the image that you are receiving heaven's force and sending that down to the person, and that you are receiving earth's force through that person and discharging it upward through your own body. You can also let your breathing follow this image, flowing up and down rather than simply in and out.

At this proceeds, the person's unbalanced vibration will gradually begin to discharge, and your hands may begin to feel numb; if this becomes too strong, wash your hands with cold water, and then resume the treatment. Then as deeper stagnation begins to dissolve and come out, you yourself may begin to feel some pain, together with a feeling of electricity; this represents the actual healing stage.

This pain will follow a certain pattern; generally, after several minutes it will begin to calm down, but may again begin to build up after several more minutes. This may repeat a number of times, with each successive buildup and calming down of pain being somewhat milder than the previous one, until finally, after a half hour or so, the pain and stagnated energy totally disappear. Aside from using your hands to send or receive energy, you can also regulate your breathing, as the following examples illustrate.

If you are treating someone with a deficient condition like anemia, have the person lie comfortably on the back and place your left hand on the center of the abdomen, in order to send energy toward the hara chakra, an important center of physical vitality. Breathe in a downward manner, with your breathing centered in the hara. When you breathe in, let your hara expand, and when you breathe out, allow it to contract. Let your exhalation become longer and slower than your inhalation. This type of breathing accelerates the flow of heaven's consolidating energy throughout your body.

If you are treating someone with an overactive condition, such as a fever, apply your right hand to the forehead, or if the fever is caused by stagnated energy in the intestines, place your right hand over the center of the abdomen. To balance the burning effect of the fever, and to accelerate the discharge of excessive energy, breathe in an upward or yin manner. To make yourself yin, keep your mouth slightly open, and make your inhalation long and slow and your exhalation short and quick. Direct the inward stream of air up toward the top of the head, rather than down toward the lungs. As you breathe in, extend your body slightly upward. Yin breathing cools the body slightly and will help the person's fever to discharge. In the course of treatment, you may yourself begin to grow warm; at the end of the treatment, it is a good idea to wash your hands and face with cold water, to completely clean yourself of the vibrations you have absorbed and helped the person discharge.

To create an overall effect of relaxation, for example, to help someone dissolve stress, and melt tension, have the person lie on his or her back and begin to stretch the person's head by gently pulling outward. Do the same for the arms and legs, and each finger and toe. Then have the person lie facing downward, preferably with the face pointing into a pillow. Begin to apply warm breath to the back of the neck in the center, while at the same time gently stroking up the back of the head toward the nose with one palm, and down the spine in the opposite direction with the other. To generate warm breath, breathe out with your mouth open and make a quiet "Huh" sound. Repeat this about three times. The combination of these techniques produces a yin or relaxing effect.

To create a yang or activating effect, have the person lie on his back and insert each of your fingers between the person's fingers of each hand and squeeze inward. Do the same for the toes on each foot. Then, have the person turn over, so that he is lying on his stomach, preferably facing downward, and begin directing cold breaths toward the back of the neck in the middle. At the same time, begin to stroke the spine in a manner opposite to the above: from the lower spine toward the neck with the palm of one hand, and from the nose toward the neck along the top and back of the head with the other. Cold breath can be generated by making a "Whew" sound. Repeat this about three times.

By applying our understanding of Kyo and Jitsu symptoms, energy-activating and energy-calming effects, and yin and yang, we can create simple palm healing treatments that are especially effective for any individual type of symptom. However, the most important conditions for effective palm healing are simply your own condition and the nature of the image and attention you hold in your mind. Let us see how these principles apply in healing specific conditions.

Healing the Eyesight

Problems with the eyes, including glaucoma and cataracts, are related to imbalance in the liver, spleen, and pancreas. In order to help heal these conditions, first treat these organs by applying your hands to the front and back of the body just below the rib cage where these organs are located. Breathe quietly for several minutes, keeping the same rhythm as the person. Then, lightly pinch the bridge of the nose with your thumb and your index or middle finger. Pinch first inward and then upward and at the same time apply your other hand to the visual center at the back of the head directly opposite the eyes. Try to coordinate the pressure applied during the pinching with your exhalation. Breathe in the same rhythm and continue for about ten minutes.

Another treatment for the eyes can be done by placing one palm over both eyes and the other on the visual center at the back of the head. Breathe along with the person, and use an upward, yin style of breathing. Continue for about ten minutes, and quickly remove your hands once you finish the treatment.

Treating Hearing Loss

The cause of hearing loss can be traced to several sources, all of which stem from the intake of improper foods. Deafness or impaired hearing can result from fat or mucus deposits in the inner ear tube, thickening of the eardrum, hardening of the delicate inner ear nerves, or blockage or stagnation along the primary channel of energy, especially around the midbrain chakra.

To help these conditions, have the person sit comfortably and from behind, cover both ears with your palms. The center of your palms should cover the earholes. Breathe together for about one minute. Insert your middle fingers into both ears and gently push inward; however, not to the extent that the person feels pain. Then, rotate your fingers with a quick, circular motion. These preliminary steps have the effect of loosening stagnation in the inner ear.

Then, with your middle fingers still inserted in the ears, begin sending vibration by making the sound of "SU." Your palms should be lightly touching the sides of the head, and for this reason, it is better to stand behind the person when giving treatment. As you sound "SU" with each exhalation, gently vibrate your middle fingers and hands. To accelerate the charge of vibration to the inner ears, the receiver can also make a sound on the exhalation. The yang, closed sound "MMM" vibrates the central regions of the nervous system, especially the midbrain chakra. After several minutes, instead of sounding "SU" on the final exhalation, direct a quick, strong breath of air to the receiver's hair spiral, making something like a "Whew" sound, while quickly removing your fingers from inside the ears. Bend over and send your breath directly to the hair spiral at a distance of about several inches.

Treating Speech Problems

Problems in the vocal cords are closely related to blockage in the flow of heaven's and earth's forces along the primary channel, especially in the throat chakra. If someone cannot speak, it is often the result of dysfunction in this main channel, since the interaction of heaven's and earth's forces is what generates the vibrations of speech. Lack of vibrating ability can also result from swollen, loose vocal cords, caused by overintake of yin foods and drinks, or from accumulation of mucus and fat in the speech mechanism.

To treat speech problems, have the person sit comfortably, and attach his tongue to the roof of his mouth, if possible, toward the back of the palate. By attaching the tongue in this manner, the flow of heaven's and earth's forces along the primary channel becomes intense. Kneel alongside the person and place one hand on the throat, so that the center of the palm covers the vocal cords. Place the tips of your thumb and middle finger in the indented area under each ear. Position your other hand above the person's head and place the middle finger of that hand lightly on the center of the person's hair spiral. Breathe together and make the sound of "SU" on the exhalation. To accelerate the healing effects of treatment, ask the receiver to make the sound "MMM" on the exhalation. Repeat ten or twelve times and suddenly release your hands. Breathe together quietly for a minute or so before concluding.

Treating Blocked Sinuses

Blocked sinuses are common today. The main cause of this condition is overintake of foods that create fat or mucus in the body, including dairy products, sugar, fruit, refined flour, and oily or greasy foods. Overconsumption of fluid can make the sinuses watery and swollen, and also contributes to blockage. To treat this condition, have the person sit comfortably while breathing in a quiet and relaxed manner. Kneel alongside the person and place one palm over the front of the face, covering the eyes, and place the other directly opposite on the back of the head. Breathe together, and make the sound "SU" on the exhalation. Ask the receiver to make the sound "MMM." After repeating several times, place the tip of your thumb and ring finger in the indented area in the center of the cheekbones on either side of the nose. Place the tip of your index or middle finger on the forehead above the nose. Keep your other hand where it is on the back of the head. Continue sounding "SU" while the receiver sounds "MMM," and repeat for several minutes. Then quickly remove your hands and return to normal breathing.

Unusual Illnesses

From time to time, persons with unusual conditions come seeking macrobiotic advice. These conditions represent imbalances in bodily energy. Below are several of these unusual cases, with an explanation of their cause according to the energetics of yin and yang, or earth's rising and heaven's descending force, and recommendations for correcting the underlying imbalance through diet and way of life.

Case 1: A young woman, about twenty-three years old, living in Portugal.

Symptoms: For about three years her head gradually began moving downward toward the right side of her body, so that it was more or less permanently pulled down toward her right shoulder. For three years she had been treated by numerous specialists. However, no positive results were produced; in other words, as far as her doctors were concerned, there was no cure for her condition. It only became worse until finally everyone gave up on her.

Cause: This is a very unusual sickness. Because of her excessive intake of strong yin foods, the right side of her body was generally more troubled. However, her left lung had become greatly expanded because of a lack of heaven's yang force. Earth's yin force was predominant in her body because of an excess of expansive energy, especially in the ascending colon.

For several years, she had been eating raw fruits and vegetables, including tropical fruits, fruit juice, and sprouts. This type of yin food caused expansion in both the lungs and intestines. Also, from consumption of dairy food, including milk, soft cheese, yogurt, and ice cream, she had developed fat and mucus deposits in the right ovary. Above her upper lip, on the right side, hair was coming out. She was growing a moustache, but only on the right side. The region of the face above the upper lip corresponds to the reproductive organs. Earth's yin, expanding force predominates in the right side of the body, while heaven's yang contracting force is stronger on the left side. If her condition were yang, then heaven's force would have pushed her head downward toward the left shoulder. Because of this, we can understand that her condition was caused by too many yin foods.

Recommendations: Even though this condition is strange, recovery is not so difficult. Of primary importance is to begin eating according to the standard macrobiotic diet, eliminating extreme foods such as sugar, fruit juice, tropical fruits, dairy and other types of animal food, and reducing the intake of raw salad. Basically, the way to recover is to bring her diet toward the center. Since her condition has been caused by extreme yin, slightly more yang methods of cooking can be used. She can include a slightly larger volume of well-cooked dishes, can eat slightly stronger miso soup, and can use condiments such as gomashio, sea vegetable powders, and others on a regular basis.

Case 2: A young man, about twenty-seven years old, living in Barcelona.

Symptoms: This young man had been suffering from a variety of strange and puzzling symptoms, including:

1. From time to time he had severe headaches.
2. He suffered from dizzy spells during which he would lose his sense of balance.
3. From time to time, he developed the urge to commit rape.
4. Very often the desire would arise in him to commit murder.
5. He masturbated heavily, as many as eight times a day.
6. He experienced frequent pain around the heart.
7. He had difficulty breathing.
8. He could not hold a job and therefore had no steady income. Although he wanted to do something, he was completely unable.
9. His eyes were very yang. Instead of the normal condition in which white is showing on either side of the iris, in his case, there was white above the iris. This condition is known as "yang sanpaku." The word "sanpaku" means "three whites." It is a sign of overall imbalance caused by too much extreme yang. During our conversation, I noticed that he blinked infrequently, another sign of an overly yang condition.

Cause: This person's original constitution was very yang from taking extreme foods such as meat, eggs, cheese, and other forms of animal fat and protein. Because of taking all these extreme yang foods when he was young, when he became a teenager, he began eating plenty of extremely yin foods, including sugar, fruit, soft drinks, and oily foods, and began using drugs. He was also taking an excess of extremely yin stimulants such as coffee, tea, black pepper, and curry powder.

His condition was caused by extremes of both yin and yang. The foods mentioned above were the cause of his disease, along with other factors. His parents' behavior was chaotic and they had separated and finally divorced. He was watching too many television shows and movies about sex and violence. All of these factors, especially his chaotic eating habits, led to his abnormal behavior and physical disorders. The organs that were most troubled were the kidneys and prostate gland. He also was suffering from hormone imbalances that were causing his sexual disorders and strange obsessions.

Recommendations: In order to restore balance, I recommended that he completely avoid foods of both extremes. For example, he should not eat meat, eggs, or cheese, and should stay away from fish or seafood until his condition improved. Similarly, he should avoid extreme yin foods or drinks, including sugar, soft drinks, and spices. The use of drugs must, of course, be stopped. I recommended that he eat according to the standard macrobiotic diet, minus fish, and include plenty of lightly cooked vegetables in his diet. An occasional raw salad or other high-quality yin, such as boiled salad or steamed greens, would also be good for healing this condition.

I further advised him to stay away from any type of violent or sex-related events, movies, or activities, and to make his surroundings as peaceful and harmonious as possible.

Case 3: A fifty-eight-year-old woman living in Caracas.
Symptoms:

1. At night, her left leg was often paralyzed or started twitching.
2. During the night, her left hip was often painful.
3. She lost hearing in her right ear.
4. Her nails had become weak and fragile.
5. Every year, during the autumn, she developed bronchitis.
6. She experienced fairly constant aches and pains around her left shoulder and back.
7. She was easily startled by loud noises.

Cause: This condition is caused extremely yin foods, especially dairy foods such as milk, cottage cheese, yogurt, and ice cream, as well as oil, sugar, and raw fruit. These extremely yin foods had produced fatty deposits in the kidneys, and also kidney stones. Oily and fatty foods, which lead to formation of mucus in the body, were especially contributing to her kidney condition.

Recommendations: Since she had been eating this way for such a long time, I suggested that she immediately stop the extreme foods that caused this unbalanced condition, and begin to eat according to the standard macrobiotic diet. One special dish recommended to help her kidney disorder was azuki beans cooked with kombu and lightly seasoned with tamari soy sauce. One small bowl, once a day, would accelerate recovery.

Case 4: Curvature of the spine that appears in many people, both male and female.

Symptoms: Around the area of the lungs the spine curves toward the right side of the body and around the large intestine it curves toward the left.

Cause: This disorder is caused by too many extreme yin foods, along with inadequate physical activity. The overconsumption of tropical fruit especially contributes to this condition, as does the overintake of sugar, dairy food, and chemically treated foods. The major organs affected are the lungs and large intestine, especially the ascending colon. The expanding effects of these extremely yin foods have caused the ascending colon to become enlarged, due to too much earth's force. This expansive energy has pushed the spine over toward the opposite side of the body.

The lungs and large intestine are complementary and antagonistic. So to make balance for this condition on the right side of the intestines, the left lung has become expanded, therefore forcing the spine over toward the right.

Recommendations: Since this condition is caused by too much yin energy in the body, we must try to make the person more yang. It is important to stop the intake of foods that are causing the condition, and have him eat according to standard macrobiotic guidelines. The following special recommendations can accelerate recovery:

1. One or two small bowls of miso soup can be eaten daily. The taste can be slightly stronger than usual, and the soup can be a little bit thicker.
2. Burdock, carrot, and other root vegetables can be eaten daily. Root vegetable dishes can be well cooked and seasoned with miso, tamari soy sauce, or sea salt.
3. The intake of liquid, including bancha tea and grain teas, should be kept at a reasonable level.
4. A person with this condition should get plenty of exercise and fresh air.

Any illness, no matter how seemingly complex, can be understood simply in terms of energy. Life is an ever-changing, moving phenomenon. Understanding the dynamics of energy enables us to orient our view in harmony with the universe and develop simple, safe, yet effective approaches to health and healing.

4
Massage and Bodywork

In a study presented at the 1989 meeting of the American Heart Association and published in *The Lancet*, Dr. Dean Ornish and associates at the University of California tested the effectiveness of diet and exercise in reversing heart disease. Twenty-two patients were placed in an experimental group and nineteen were assigned to a control group. All of the patients were suffering from severe coronary blockage. Patients in the experimental group ate a diet based on whole grains, beans, and vegetables with less than 10 percent fat, took daily half-hour walks, and practiced meditation, stretching, and breathing exercises twice a week. The members of the control group did not practice stress reduction and most ate a less balanced diet of about 30 percent fat.

The difference between the two groups was striking. After one year, eighteen of the experimental patients showed significant unblocking of the arteries. Three experienced slight unblocking, and one patient, who did not comply with the program, showed progression of the condition. The experimental patients also experienced a 91 percent reduction in the frequency of chest pains, a 42 percent reduction in their duration, and a 28 percent reduction in their severity. In contrast, ten of the nineteen patients in the control group experienced progression of their disease. On the whole, the control group experienced an increase in the frequency, duration, and severity of chest pains.

Activity and movement are essential components of a healthful lifestyle. Walking, for example, activates the flow of energy in the chakras, meridians, and throughout the body. It also stimulates circulation, improves breathing, tones the muscles, and increases appetite. Because it stimulates breathing and circulation, walking helps cleanse the blood. The added oxygen in the blood oxidizes (burns) impurities, and the lymphatic system, which carries wastes from the cells, also cleanses itself. Walking also clears the mind and dissolves stress, and reduces the risk of chronic illness.

A study published in the *Journal of the American Medical Association* in November 1989 concluded that moderate exercise, including a brisk half-hour walk every day, reduced the risk of cancer and heart disease. The researchers discovered that people who exercise moderately tend to live longer, and the study added to the evidence that exercise can help prevent cancer, a relationship discovered only in the past several years. Exercise helps increase bowel motility, a factor that helps prevent colon cancer.

In this chapter, we present a variety of practices that can help improve circulation, energize the meridians and chakras, clear the mind, and reduce stress, beginning with the traditional, holistic practice of shiatsu, or "finger-pressure," massage.

Massage

Massage is one of the most important elements of holistic healing. Like acupuncture, moxibustion, and palm healing, it involves stimulating and unblocking the meridians and points along which electromagnetic energy, or Ki, flows throughout the body. Energy flow becomes blocked or stagnated through accumulation of mucus, fats, or toxins in the blood, organs, or joints, which in turn causes stiffness or pain along the meridians. These blockages and accumulations are caused by dietary imbalances and a lack of proper activity. These blockages interfere with the flow of energy along the meridians and can contribute to illness.

Basic massage uses only the hands and fingertips and can be learned in several hours. With practice, the student can develop his or her ability and make massage into a comprehensive and effective healing art. It can be done almost anytime and anywhere.

The style of massage presented below is based on a deep understanding of the energy constitution of the body, and the interconnectedness of all of its parts and functions. Shiatsu deals with underlying energy imbalances and helps improve overall vitality and conductivity to the forces of heaven and earth. In this way, it helps activate overall vitality and conductivity to environmental energy.

Making your energy harmonious with that of the person you are treating is an intrinsic element of massage. It is therefore important to remember that the physical condition of the practitioner is a key factor in its success. Someone who is healthy, eats a diet of whole grains and vegetables, and who radiates a calm and vibrant energy will transfer this to the person who is receiving the massage.

The basic full-body massage can be simplified in five stages: (1) the shoulders, neck, and head; (2) the back; (3) the arms and hands; (4) the legs and feet; and (5) the front of the body. The basic massage routine presented below can be adapted to each person's needs and condition. If, for example, a person is experiencing pain or severe rigidity in the joints or in any other part of the body, it is advisable to omit the procedures that call for massaging these areas. You can try the full body massage presented below, one step at a time, or can try only parts of it.

Also, unlike other forms of massage, shiatsu does not require the removal of clothing or the use of oils. Loose-fitting cotton is best for giving and receiving massage. The massage can also be performed simply on blankets or cushions placed on the floor. For complete diagrams of the meridians and points referred to below, see my books, *Macrobiotics and Oriental Medicine* and *The Book of Do-In*, published by Japan Publications, Inc.

Shoulders

If the shoulders are tight, swollen, and painful when pressed, energy is not flowing smoothly through the body. A person in this condition has difficulty relaxing and is frequently tired. Tight shoulders are also a sign of stagnation in the intestines that blocks the active flow of energy in the hara and sexual chakras, diminishing the vitality and functioning of the organs in the lower body.

To help relieve shoulder tension, release intestinal stagnation, and vitalize the flow of energy in the body as a whole:

1. Have the person sit comfortably with his or her spine straight and shoulders and arms relaxed. Keeping your spine straight, kneel behind the person. Extend your arms forward and grasp both shoulders with a firm but gentle pressure. Keep your hands in this position and begin to harmonize your energies by breathing together. (This will help the person relax and make him or her receptive to the massage.) With your hands in this position, breathe together for about a minute.

2. Begin to massage the shoulders with a kneading motion. Start with the area closest to the neck and gradually work outward toward the tips of the shoulders. Repeat several times.

3. Stand up behind the person. Keeping your thumbs straight, press with the tips of both thumbs along the top of the shoulder muscles on both sides of the neck. Gently push in, and then quickly release the pressure. Begin from the innermost region on both sides of the neck, and work outward toward the tips of the shoulders.

When performing this part of the massage, coordinate your breathing with that of the person. To do this properly, inhale together, and as you breathe out, press downward. Press along the shoulder muscle several times before proceeding to the next step of the massage.

4. With your hands in the position indicated in step one, extend your middle fingers down the front of the body to massage

the area under the collarbone on both sides. Using the tips of the fingers, massage for about one minute. If this area is painful or overly sensitive, the lungs are overexpanded from mucus deposits, liquids, and sugar.

5. Keeping your wrists loose and flexible, use the outside edge of your hands to gently pound the shoulders by rapidly alternating between the left and right hand. Begin at the neck and work your way outward. The shoulders can be done separately or both at the same time. Repeat several times. After finishing step five, again massage the shoulders as in step two.

Neck

Tension or stiffness in the neck is a common problem today, aggravated by the overconsumption of protein, saturated fat, sugar, refined foods, and overeating and overdrinking in general.

When the neck becomes stiff, energy does not flow smoothly through the small intestine, large intestine, stomach, bladder, and gallbladder meridians, all of which run along the neck. Stiffness in the neck also indicates diminished physical and mental flexibility, including a reduced capacity for natural, spontaneous expression and enjoyment.

To help relieve tension in the neck and stimulate the flow of energy to the organs and along those meridians:

1. Shift your position so that you are sitting behind the person at a 45-degree angle. Place the bulk of your weight on one knee and raise your other leg so that your foot is on the floor. If you are right-handed, shift to the left, so that you can use your left hand to support the person's forehead, while leaving your right hand free to massage the back of the neck. Persons who are left-handed should shift in the opposite direction, leaving the left hand free for the neck massage.

2. Tilt the person's head slightly backward, and place the tips of your thumb and middle finger in the indented places at the base of the skull on both sides of the back of the neck. Massage

this region for about a minute or until hardness or tension is relieved. Pain in this area frequently indicates that the person is eating too many fatty foods, which interfere with the smooth functioning of the liver and gallbladder.

3. Return the person's head to the normal angle, and beginning from the above regions, use the tip of your thumb and middle finger to massage in a straight line down the back of the neck to the base. (Use a deep but gentle pinching motion in which you knead and stimulate the neck muscle with your fingertips.) Repeat several times, making sure to loosen any hardness or tension.

4. Place the tip of your thumb in the center of the neck at the base of the skull. Begin breathing together, and after several breaths, tilt the head back, as in step two, and on the final inhalation, push your thumb inward and upward into the point, lifting the head slightly upward. (Use your supporting hand to help lift the head.) At the peak of the inhalation, vibrate your thumb for several seconds, and as you breathe out, release the pressure and allow the head to return to its normal position. Repeat several times.

5. Return to your original position behind the person. Place your right hand firmly on the shoulder, resting the inside of the hand against the neck for support. With your left hand on the left side of the head, begin to rotate the head slowly toward the right in a clockwise direction. (This helps relax tension in the neck and shoulders.) As much as possible, allow the head to rotate itself; it is better to use your hands only to support and guide the rotation. After a minute, reverse your hands and begin to rotate in the opposite, counterclockwise direction. (This helps to stabilize the flow of energy in the person's body.) Continue for about one minute.

Head

In the human body and throughout nature, the part reflects the whole. This is especially true in the relationship between the head and the rest of the body, since there are areas on the head that relate to all of the major organs and body functions, including the chakras.

To stimulate these areas and their corresponding organs and functions, and energize the body as a whole:

1. Stand up behind the person. Place your fingers on either side of his or her head and extend your thumbs so that they are free to massage the central part of the top of the head. Place your thumbs behind each other, and press down in a straight line extending from the hairline back across the top of the head and down the back of the head to the base of the skull. Repeat several times.

2. Directly on top of the head in the center is a point known in Oriental countries as the "hundred meeting point." Energy from all over the body gathers there. Place your fingers on either side of the receiver's head and position your thumbs just above the point. Breathe together several times, and at the peak of the final exhalation, press the hundred meeting point. While applying pressure, vibrate your thumbs for several seconds and then release. This helps to release energy that has become stagnant anywhere in the body. Repeat several times.

3. Locate the person's hair spiral. Position your hands as in step two, breathe together, and press your thumbs into the center of the spiral, using the same methods as above. Release and repeat several times. The hair spiral is the place where heaven's force enters the body, and from here, flows down along the primary channel. Massaging the hair spiral helps to energize and vitalize the flow of energy in the chakras and body as a whole.

4. Extend your fingers down the sides of the head, and with your middle fingers, massage both temples simultaneously, using a slow, upward circular motion. Continue for about a minute or until all tension in this area is released.

5. Grasp both ears with thumbs and middle fingers. Begin to massage the ears by pulling them gently upward from the top, outward from the side, and then downward from the lobe. Repeat several times, allowing your fingers to slide across the inner por-

tion of the ear to the edge. The ears correlate with the kidneys, and this part of the massage is good for loosening stagnation in these organs and improving overall vitality.

6. Using your fingertips, gently pound the top of the head, making sure to keep your wrists loose and flexible. (You can also tighten your hands into a fist and gently pound the head with your knuckles.) Be sure to stimulate the entire head, including the top, sides, and back. Do each region for about thirty seconds.

After finishing this part of the massage, sit down behind the person and again knead the shoulders as explained previously. If the massage has been done properly, the shoulders should be soft and relaxed, meaning that the flow of energy along the primary channel, chakras, and meridians is now smooth and active.

The Back

Massaging the back stimulates the flow of energy through all of the major organs. This is accomplished by massaging the bladder meridian (running along either side of the spine), the chakras, and the roots of the autonomic nerve branches (radiating outward from the spinal cord to the internal organs). The bladder meridian includes points where energy from the atmosphere enters the body and charges each of the major organs.

To energize these organs and functions:

1. Have the person lie on his or her stomach, the head turned sideways and arms extended comfortably to the side.

2. Kneel alongside the person so that one hand is free to massage the entire back. If you are right-handed, sit on their left; vice versa if you are left-handed. Place your hand so that the center of the palm rests lightly on the spine. Slowly brush down the spine to the buttocks, as if you were smoothing the flow of energy downward.

3. Place one palm on the spine, and place your other hand on top of it. Starting at the upper spine, breathe together, and as you

exhale, gently press downward. Add your body weight by leaning forward as you press. Release pressure during the next inhalation, and repeat down the length of the spine to the tailbone.

4. To massage the meridian running along the center of the
spine (which energizes the chakras), insert your thumbs one below the other in the indented spaces between the vertebrae. Extend your fingers outward and place them on the rib cage for support. Begin at the top of the spine. Breathe together and on the
exhalation gently push your thumbs inward, releasing pressure
on the following inhalation. Insert your thumbs in the next set of
spaces and repeat down the entire length of the spine.

5. Hold your fingers firmly together and extend them outward. Insert your fingertips in the indented area on either side of
the spine. Beginning at the upper spine, move your hand rapidly
in a cutting or sawing motion. Work your way down the entire
length of the spine, using this indented area as a pathway. Do the
same thing on the opposite side of the spine.

6. Find the inner set of bladder meridians which run along
two parallel lines located about two finger widths out from the
center of the spine. Using the technique described above, press
your thumbs along the length of the meridian, beginning at the
shoulders and proceeding down the back and across the buttocks
in one-inch steps. When massaging the rib cage, insert your
thumbs in the spaces between the ribs. To send energy through
the points and to the corresponding organs, as you press each
point, rotate the tip of your thumbs in a counterclockwise direction. To release energy from the points and corresponding organs, rotate your thumbs in a clockwise direction.

7. Find the outer set of bladder meridians which run along
two parallel lines about two finger widths out from the inner set
of meridians. Use the above technique to massage both sides simultaneously, from the shoulders to the buttocks.

8. Use the fingertips, thumb, and base of the palm to massage the receiver's shoulder blade. Continue with active massage
for about one minute, loosening any tension in the surrounding
muscles and tendons. Repeat with the other shoulder blade.

9. Place your thumb in the center of the shoulder blade.

Breathe together with the receiver, and press as you exhale, massaging this area with a quick circular motion. Repeat three times and proceed to the other shoulder blade. Rotate your thumb counterclockwise to send energy; clockwise to release energy from the receiver's body.

10. Place both hands together across the spine in the region of the waist. Place your thumbs on one side, and your fingers on the other side of the spine. Use a deep kneading motion to massage this area. Pain here is a sign of expansion or tightness in the kidneys, and indicates potential weakening of overall vitality.

11. Use your palm, fingers, and thumb to knead and rub the entire back, relieving any tension or stagnation in the muscles and along the meridians. Start at the upper region and massage down the periphery of the back, one side at a time. Use your left hand to send energy to the receiver; your right hand to draw energy from the receiver's body. After you finish, smooth the flow of energy down the spine and both sides of the back.

12. To massage the buttocks, move slightly downward so that you can reach the indented area in the center of both sides of the buttock. Push the base of your palms firmly in this area and then massage with an upward and outward circular motion. Repeat for about one minute. This is especially good for strengthening overall vitality. Then, place your hand on the tailbone. Use the base of your palm to gently pound the tailbone. Continue for about thirty seconds, in order to send stimulation along the entire length of the spine.

The Arms and Hands

Six meridians run along the arm. Three—the lung, heart governor (the comprehensive body function responsible for the circulation of blood and body fluids), and heart—run down the inside of the arm from the armpit to the hand, and out to the fingers. The other three—the large intestine, triple heater (the body-wide function responsible for the generation of heat and caloric energy), and small intestine—run from the fingers up the outside of the arm to the shoulder. Each of the fingers, with the exception of the little finger, has one meridian. The little finger has two meridians, the heart and small intestine. This pattern is a reflection of the process in which one cell divides into two, two into four, four into eight, and so on, and the process by which a husband and wife produce children, children produce grandchildren, and so on through time. The process in which one divides into two, two into four, four into eight, and so on endlessly is described by Lao Tsu in the *Tao Teh Ching*. It describes the process in which the universe and all phenomena come into being.

In the human body, there are three basic divisions: (1) front and back, (2) up and down, and (3) left and right. The process of division continues within the hand as the thumb separates from the fingers in stage (4). In the next stage (5), the fingers divide into two groups, the index and middle fingers, and the ring and little fingers. The two groups then separate into individual fingers in the next stage (6). In the final stage (7), the little finger divides into two meridians, thus completing a seven-staged process of growth and development. To massage the arms and hands:

1. Place your hand on the root of the arm with your thumb inserted in the person's armpit and your fingers placed across the top of the shoulder joint. Grasp the wrist with your other hand and stretch the arm by pushing your hand down and gently pulling the arm outward with your other hand. Repeat several times.

2. Grasp the arm by placing both hands in the area between the wrist and the elbow. Using the shoulder as the axis of rotation, gently twist the entire arm first in one direction and then in the other. Repeat several times.

3. Place one hand above and the other below the elbow. Gently twist the upper and lower sections of the arm in opposite directions, as if you were wringing out a wet towel. Repeat by twisting each section in the reverse direction.

4. Use the palm and fingers of your active hand to press down both sides of the arm, loosening any tension in the muscles and tendons. Work your way down to the hands and fingertips.

5. Imagine three parallel lines running about 1/4 of an inch apart along the inside of the arm from the armpit to the wrist. These correspond roughly to the heart, heart governor, and lung meridians. Place one hand under the arm for support, and with the thumb of your other hand, press along each line, starting at the armpit and working your way down to the wrist. First, massage the heart meridian, then the heart governor, and finally the lung meridian. As you massage down each line, spend extra time massaging the elbow and wrist portion with a gentle circular thumb motion.

6. As with the above step, imagine three parallel lines running along the outside of the arm, this time in the opposite direction from the wrist to the shoulder. These lines correspond roughly to the large intestine, triple heater, and small intestine meridians. Using the same technique, massage down these outer lines from the wrist to the shoulder. Start with the large intestine and proceed to the triple heater and small intestine meridians.

7. Support the person's wrist with one hand, and with the other, gently rotate the hand several times. Repeat in the opposite direction.

8. Place the hand on one knee for support. Position the little finger of one of your hands between the thumb and index finger of the person's hand, and position your other little finger between the ring and little fingers. Using your little fingers for support, massage the palms by rapidly pressing your thumbs one after the other into the palm, working your way around the entire hand. Place special emphasis on the area adjacent to the thumb which corresponds to the digestive and respiratory systems.

Pain or a reddish or bluish color in this area indicate possible swelling or fatty deposits in the intestines. Massage the center of both palms. This area, which is a part of the heart governor meridian, energizes the heart, stomach, and hara chakras, together with sexual vitality. Pain in this point frequently indicates that the heart and circulatory system is overworking, and that a person may be experiencing overall fatigue. Place one hand under the person's hand for support, and with the thumb of your active hand, press the center of the palm, and then release. To send energy, rotate your thumb in a counterclockwise direction. To release energy, rotate your thumb clockwise. Repeat several times.

9. Turn the hand so that the outside is exposed. Find the indented area between the thumb and index finger. Massage this area for about one minute, using a deep, circular thumb motion to release tension and stagnation. This area is along the large intestine meridian. Pain or tightness indicate stagnation or overexpansion in the large intestine.

10. Each of the fingers corresponds to one of the meridians which run along the arm, in the following order: thumb—lung; index finger—large intestine; middle finger—heart governor; ring finger—triple heater; little finger (inside)—heart; and little finger (outside)—small intestine.

When massaging the fingers, imagine a series of five points, three located in the center of the three sections of each finger and two located immediately below the finger on the palm. (Use four points when massaging the thumb—two in the center of each section and two immediately below in the root of the thumb.) Grasp the wrist with one hand and turn the palm upward. Massage each finger separately by pressing each point with the tip of your thumb, rotating your thumb in a circular motion, releasing, and then proceeding to the next point. (Start with the points located at the root of the fingers. To send energy to the meridians, rotate your thumb counterclockwise; to release energy, rotate your thumb clockwise. Place your fingers on the opposite side of each finger for support.) When you reach the last point on the tip of each finger, pull and rotate the finger several times.

11. Use your palm and fingers to brush down both sides of the arm and out through the fingertips. Repeat several times.

Shift to the other side of the person and massage the other arm in the above steps.

The Legs and Feet

The bladder, gallbladder, and stomach meridians run down along the back, sides, and front of the leg. The kidney, spleen, and liver meridians run up along the inside. Of primary importance when massaging the legs is to activate the flow of energy along these meridian pathways.

To massage the legs:

1. Have the person lie on his stomach. Shift your position so that you are below his feet. In most cases, you will notice that the legs are not perfectly even. If one leg is longer than the other, this indicates a degree of imbalance between the right and left sides of the body. It may also indicate that the pelvis is slanted in the direction of the longer leg; the result of overexpansion in the organs located on that side, especially lower organs like the kidneys, intestines, and sexual organs.

To help correct this imbalance, grasp the shorter leg below the ankle. Gently pull the leg slightly upward and outward, lower it to the ground, and then release.

2. Grasp both feet by holding the toes between your palms and fingers. Bend the leg at the knee, cross the feet at the ankles, and press them backward into the buttocks. If the legs and feet are painful or not flexible enough to do this, do not force them.

With the legs in this position, reverse the feet and again press down into the buttocks. After you finish, return the feet to their normal position on the floor.

3. The bladder meridian, which runs down the back, continues down the back of both legs in the center and out to the fifth toe. Using the thumb, press down the meridian from the buttock to the ankle. (Each leg may be massaged separately or both at the same time.) Use a gentle, penetrating pressure when massaging this meridian; however, ease up when you reach the sensitive area behind the knee, as pressure here can be painful. If the receiver feels pain when you press the part of the meridian on the center of the calf (corresponding to the large intestine), his or her

intestines are overexpanded, and energy in the hara chakra has become weak.

4. Raise one leg by bending it at the knee. Place one hand below the ankle and grasp the toes with the other. Begin to rotate the foot in a circular motion for about one minute in one direction and then in the other. Do not force the foot to rotate beyond the point at which discomfort is experienced. Pain or lack of flexibility in the ankles is a sign of hardening of the arteries and joints, and of a general decline in conductivity to heaven's and earth's forces.

5. With the leg in the above position, use one hand to press the foot downward so that it is parallel to the floor. With the thumb and index finger of your other hand, massage the Achilles tendon by rubbing it vigorously up and down. This tendon corresponds to the sexual organs. It should be tight and somewhat firm. If it is loose, the sexual organs may have become weak as a result of dietary excess. A coating of fat around the Achilles tendon also suggests fat and mucus deposits in the sexual organs. Massage the Achilles tendon for about thirty seconds. This helps energize sexual vitality.

6. Keeping the foot in the above position, locate the region on the inside of the leg about four finger widths up from the ankle. Known in Japanese as the "junction of three yin meridians," this area corresponds with the spleen, liver, and kidneys. This region was used traditionally by Oriental doctors to treat disorders in the sexual organs but should not be massaged when a woman is pregnant. Use the thumb of your free hand to massage this region for about thirty seconds with a deep but gentle circular motion.

7. Actively massage the bottom of the foot by alternately pressing with the fingers of your left and right hands. (Place your thumbs opposite to your fingers on the underside of the foot for support.) Massage the entire sole of the foot for about thirty seconds in this manner.

8. On the bottom of the foot, about three fingers below the junction of the second and third toes, is an important point on the kidney meridian. Known in Japanese as "bubbling spring," this

point is where energy in the kidney meridian begins its course up the inside of the leg. Place your free hand on the opposite side of the foot for support and press the point with your thumb. (You may also vibrate your thumb as you are applying pressure.) Release pressure and repeat several times. If this point is overly sensitive or painful, the kidneys are not functioning at their optimum. To send energy to the kidneys, massage this point in a counterclockwise motion. To release energy from the kidneys, use a clockwise motion. Thickening of the skin on the kidney point is caused by overintake of animal protein and fat and indicates that energy is not flowing smoothly along the kidney meridian, and that overall vitality is below par.

9. Massage the toes by using the pinching technique described for the fingers. As with the fingers, work your way outward to the tip, and then pull and rotate each toe. When you finish each toe, pull excess energy out by gently pulling and snapping the tip.

Each toe corresponds to a particular organ and meridian in the following order: large toe (outside)—spleen; large toe (inside)—liver; second and third toes—stomach; fourth toe—gallbladder; fifth toe—bladder. Each of these organs and their corresponding meridians are stimulated and activated when we massage the toes.

10. Supporting the foot from the underside, use your free hand to rapidly pound the entire bottom of the foot. (Tighten your fingers into a fist and pound with the side of your hand.) Like the head, palms, ears, and back, the bottoms of the feet correspond to the entire body, and the entire body benefits when we stimulate them.

After you finish the above steps, lower the foot to the floor and repeat steps four through ten with the other foot. After massaging both feet, brush the person's energy down both legs from the buttocks to the toes.

The Front of the Body

Of primary importance when massaging the front of the body is to stimulate the front organs directly along with the leg meridians. These include the kidney, spleen, and liver meridians which run up the inside of the leg, and the stomach and gallbladder meridians which run down the front side. As this is a basic technique, just massage in the general vicinity of the meridians, rather than trying to locate them precisely or to identify specific points. To energize these meridians and organs:

1. Have the person turn over so that he or she is lying comfortably on the back. Grasp both legs by the ankles and massage upward to the pelvis, generally loosening any tension in the muscles. Repeat this several times.

2. Imagine three parallel lines running up the inside of the leg from the ankle to the pelvis. These correspond roughly to the kidney, spleen, and liver meridians. Place your fingers on the outside of the leg for support, and press upward along each line with your thumbs. Each leg can be massaged separately or both at the same time.

3. Imagine a line running down the top of the leg on the outside of the knee from the pelvis to the foot. This generally corresponds to the stomach meridian. Keep your hands in the position described above, only this time, use your fingers to massage down the line and your thumb for support. The legs can be massage one at a time or simultaneously.

4. Imagine a line running down the outside of the leg from the hip socket to the foot. This corresponds roughly to the gallbladder meridian. Using the above technique, massage down this line also.

5. Have the person raise his or her knees and place the feet flat on the floor. Place your hands on the knees and press the knees upward and then downward toward the abdomen. This helps release tension deep within the intestines. Return the legs to their resting position on the floor.

6. Place the fingers of your active hand together and extend them firmly outward. Place the tips of your extended fingers on the lower right side of the abdomen in the region of the ascending colon. Breathe together and on the exhalation, press gently into the abdomen. Release pressure with the following exhalation, and reposition your hand further up along the ascending colon. Repeat this procedure along the entire length of the colon, moving across the transverse colon and then down the descending colon on the left side.

Pain or hardness in the large intestine is a sign of mucus and fat accumulations, or swelling due to the overintake of saturated fats, flour products, sugar, liquid, and overeating in general. This practice can be repeated several times as it is good for promoting regularity in the bowels and releasing stagnation in the lower body.

7. Place your hands across the abdomen. Begin to gently knead and massage the small intestine. Continue for about a minute.

8. Place your thumbs under the rib cage. Breathe together and on the exhalation gently press inward and upward. This step is good for activating the liver, spleen, pancreas, and stomach. Repeat several times.

9. To complete the massage, place one hand lightly on the person's abdomen and the other lightly on the forehead. Breathe together for a minute or two, or until he or she is completely relaxed. Detach your hands by raising them slowly upward.

Conclusion

If the massage has been done properly, your partner should feel relaxed yet energized. After you complete the massage, ask the person to remain in a resting position for about five minutes. Meanwhile, wash your hands in cold water to remove any excess energy that you may have picked up during the massage. With this, your basic massage is now complete.

Once the basic massage technique has been mastered, feel

free to experiment and continuously add new approaches to your practice. In this way, your massage will remain dynamic, and you will be able to develop your own original style.

Each massage will always be slightly different. The basic routine can serve as a general outline; however, it needs to be flexibly adapted to suit the needs of every person whom you treat. For example, in the morning or during the day, an active, stimulating massage is usually appropriate, while in the evening, a relaxing or calming massage would be more suitable.

Similarly, you would massage a child differently than an elderly person, and a man slightly differently than a woman. Also, since everyone's condition is unique, it is important to develop your diagnostic ability. In this way, you can adjust your massage to suit the needs of the person you are treating. When you develop this intuitive ability and use it in conjunction with a centered, orderly technique, you are on your way to becoming a compassionate healer.

As we saw in Chapter 2, the meridians serve as channels for consciousness and emotion. When we stimulate them, we produce an effect on the mind and emotions, and on the physical functioning of the organs and body as a whole. Massaging the fingers and toes will produce a corresponding effect on the mental and emotional functions connected with each meridian. Stimulating the lung meridian, for example, by massaging the thumb, activates the person's intellect. Stimulating the right thumb has a mildly activating effect, while stimulating the left thumb has a strong activating effect. If we send energy to the large intestine by massaging the index finger, we make it easier for the person to become centered and establish order and stability in his social relations. Stimulating the right thumb produces a mildly stabilizing effect, while stimulating the left thumb has a strongly stabilizing effect. Similar relationships exist on each finger and toe.

Through massage, we can either activate and energize a person's thoughts and emotions, or stabilize and quiet them down. Shiatsu helps us to establish harmony between body and mind, physical and energetic functions, and visible and invisible aspects of our being.

Do-In

Unlike Western medicine, Oriental medicine is not analytical. It is holistic and comprehensive, and might more properly be called a way of life. It involves cosmology, mentality, and daily life, though we can specify five medical arts:

1. Selection and preparation of daily food
2. Acupuncture, including moxibustion, massage, and shiatsu
3. Natural herbs and minerals
4. Do-In
5. Surgery

Do-In consists of exercises or practices (such as meditation or chanting) that bring out hidden potentialities of health and energy from the body. Although it is still practiced in China, Do-In has all but died out in Japan. When Western medicine came to Japan, people were amazed by its organized analytical methods. Soon the government and leaders decreed that all doctors must study Western medicine. At that time, they also examined all traditional methods of healing and licensed some methods to continue as unofficial medicine. Acupuncture, food, and herbal medicine were allowed to remain. There are still stores that sell only traditional recipes for herbs, but by and large, drugstores sell only Western drugs. Because people had already forgotten yin and yang they could not understand Do-In. As a result, it was not sanctioned. Surgery was developed as long as three thousand years ago, by a doctor named Kada. He used an herbal tonic that put people to sleep and then he could perform surgical operations, including delicate brain surgery.

Although Do-In has more or less disappeared because people could not justify or explain its practices according to modern science, we can still present some of these techniques, several of which have been known and used for thousands of years.

1. To stop hiccoughing, press and rub the center of the palms. Pain indicates that the muscles of the upper chest are tensed and hardened. These muscles control the diaphragm, which in turn regulates breathing.

2. To clear stuffed nostrils, grab the toes of the corresponding nostril (left foot for the left side of the nose) and pull outward. Then thoroughly rub the top and bottom of the toes. Another technique is to close your eyes and walk backward slowly without bending the knees. If you cannot balance properly, it shows that the stuffed nose is harming your sense of balance.

3. For headaches in the front or sides of the head, clamp the nostrils with your fingers and pull down, but continue to breathe through the mouth. At the same time, move the eyes from right to left. This eye movement, plus stopping the nose, is more yang; the midbrain is yangized, helping to make balance with these yin types of headaches.

4. Motion sickness, sea sickness, or a general feeling of nausea in the stomach can be relieved by interlocking the little fingers of each hand and pulling. This yang action cancels the yin upward motion of vomiting.

5. When the heartbeat is faster than normal, apply the heel of the hand to each closed eye and push hard, but gently, on the eyeball. First use pressure on one and then the other eye. Another technique is to pull hard on the middle finger of both hands. Powerfully pulling then massaging the big toe is also effective.

6. For kidney trouble, close the eyes and simultaneously hit the backs of each ear with the fingers. Continue this way for about twenty or thirty times. Another technique is to place the hand over the ear and strike it with two crossed fingers. The sound created stimulates the kidneys. If that sound causes pain, the nerve of the inner ear is swollen from excessive liquid.

7. There are many techniques of Do-In used for the liver. One is to press up underneath the bottom of the rib cage. Although the liver is on the right side, use fingers on both sides. Another way to stimulate the liver is by rubbing the two large toes of each foot together. This activates the whole body. Also one can rotate the large toes about fifty times in each direction.

There is a close connection between the liver and the eyes. Rub the palms until they are hot and cover the eyes. Leaving the eyes open, move them up and down and then right to left, approximately thirty times.

8. To stimulate the pancreas, sit on the heels in the Japanese fashion, then sit up straight, extending the legs at the thighs. At the same time bring the arms to the stomach and exhale deeply, hitting the stomach.

9. For intestine trouble, vigorously rub the area between the thumb and index finger on the outside of both hands. You can also massage the calf. Bang the top of the head with one hand, then the other, first straight down from the top and then at a forty-five degree angle. For relief of constipation, about two hundred times is good. Walking barefoot on stones also stimulates the intestines.

10. To improve digestion in the stomach, pull up on the ears, and raise the entire body. Also, rubbing the nose up and down is good.

11. Through our understanding of physiognomy, we know that the lungs are related to the cheeks. If the lungs are weak, rub the hands together until warm and then rub the cheeks. Rubbing the inside ridge of the ear is also effective.

12. For a general increase in vitality or sexual appetite, have a friend repeatedly press down and slowly release the spiral at the top of the head. Or massage just to the rear and slightly below the waist bone, toward the rear of the body. Pain here indicates deterioration of the kidneys and reproductive organs.

13. The principle behind Do-In is good circulation. To increase circulation generally, rub or pull the outside of the ear or cheeks. By rubbing the fingers until warm and covering the nose and mouth, circulation will be increased. Hop on the toes. In other words, treat the periphery of the body in some way.

If you suffer from nervous tension, which means that the autonomic nervous system is out of balance, close the eyes and walk backward. By reversing the customary muscle movements, the tendency of the entire body is reversed. In the case of mental instability there is another method: rub the spine simply and slowly until it is warm, just like patting a dog. At the end, slow down until stopping. The person's mentality will become still and quiet.

There are many techniques in Do-In, but the most basic one for longevity and keeping young is rubbing the hands and feet. In the East, this is called the "method of longevity." All other methods are subsidiary to it. Some of them can be understood easily; others require a deep understanding of yin and yang, physiognomy, and the meridians. We use many of them every day without knowing it. They are all based on the energetic relationships found throughout the human body and help maintain health and vitality.

Body Scrubbing

Scrubbing your body with a moist, hot towel is a wonderfully natural way to energize your vitality, relieve stress, and relax tension. It is similar to Do-In and takes only about ten minutes to do.

Body scrubbing can be done before or after a bath or shower, or anytime. All you need is a sink with hot water and a medium-sized cotton bath towel. Turn on the hot water. Hold the towel at either end and place the center of the towel under the stream of hot water. Wring out the towel, and while it is still hot and steamy, begin to scrub with it. Do a section of the body at a time. For example, begin with the hands and fingers and work your way up the arms to the shoulders, neck, and face, then down to the chest, upper back, abdomen, lower back, buttocks, legs, feet, and toes. Scrub until the skin turns slightly red or until each part becomes warm. Reheat the towel by running it under hot water after doing each section or as soon as it starts to cool.

The body scrub releases blockage and allows environmental energy to flow smoothly through the body. In the morning, atmospheric energy moves in an outward and upward direction, producing the tendency toward physical activity. In the evening, atmospheric energy moves downward and inward, producing the tendency toward mental activity, along with physical relaxation and rest. Body scrubbing keeps us in touch with the natural coming and going, waxing and waning, upward and downward flow of energy in the atmosphere. A morning body scrub has the effect of activating energy flow and vitality. When done in the evening, a body scrub calms and relaxes us, melting and dissolving tension and stress. Moreover, scrubbing with a hot towel helps melt deposits of hard fat just below the skin, increasing its sensitivity to energy in the environment and energizing the meridians, organs, and chakras.

Foot Soaking

Overconsumption of meat, chicken, eggs, cheese, and other animal products frequently leads to the formation of thick, hard skin on the bottoms of the feet and toes. These formations represent the discharge of excessive protein and saturated fat, and interfere with the smooth flow of energy in the body. As we saw above, each toe is part of a meridian that energizes a major organ. Moreover, certain points or locations on the bottom of the foot correspond to different parts of the body. The art of foot reflexology is based on these correspondences.

Soaking the feet helps soften these hardened deposits and allows energy to flow smoothly through the meridians. Simply fill the bathtub with enough hot water to cover your feet. Place both feet in the tub and soak for about five minutes until they become red or warm. This can be done every evening before bed to relax your body and to establish an active energy flow through the meridians and chakras. Walking barefoot on the beach, soil, or grass is also an excellent way to charge your meridians and chakras with energy.

5
Dimensions of Diagnosis

Everything exists in the present, including the past and future. Our present condition represents our past eating, together with our future sickness or health. Our body, our face, our palms represent our whole past and our whole future. As you know, your future can change. The past is already past, and it is accumulated as the present condition. So our present condition reflects our past, and therefore naturally our future direction. But we can change the future if we so wish. In order to do that we must change our present way of eating and living.

Everyone's present condition contains strengths and weaknesses. No one has all good points or all bad points. We are a mixture of both. We can all be improved. Let us begin our study of diagnosis with a review of facial characteristics, starting with the head.

Head

When evaluating a person's constitution, one of the first things to note is the shape of the head. Generally speaking there are four types of head shapes—square, triangular with the top expanded, triangular with the bottom expanded, and round. The triangular shape with the expansion on the bottom is the most yang. The triangular shape with the expansion at the top is the most yin. This type of person will probably like poetry, art, and music. A square face is also yang, but not as yang as a face with the shape of a pyramid. A round shaped face is also yang, but not to the extent of a square face.

If the back of the head is large and expanded, it shows the tendency toward violent or criminal behavior. Expansion of the back of the head indicates that the cerebellum is enlarged. This part of the brain should be small. It controls activity and action. If the cerebellum is swollen, it indicates that there will be too much action—thus the potential for violent behavior.

The shape of the head can be changed when the person is still a baby. If someone is born with a swollen cerebellum, this condition can be corrected by eating good food during the first few years of life. The head will change its shape and the baby's personality will also change. By this we can understand that criminal tendencies are not necessarily inherited. Rather they are the result of the food we eat. Any criminal person can be changed into an honest one by changing the pattern of food intake.

Hair

There are many things we can see by looking at the hair. For example, the hair shows the condition of the intestinal villi. There are millions of villi in the intestinal tract. Just as the head is the compact form of the rest of the body, so the hair on the head reflects the intestinal villi. When we look at the condition of the hair, we can immediately see the condition of the intestinal villi. The health of the intestinal villi shows the power of the person's digestion. Therefore when we see the a person's hair, we can tell what his digestive ability is.

The villi are tiny and compact. Therefore the hair on the head is larger and more expanded. The nature of the villi and the hair is the same, but they are the opposite of each other. The villi are yang, while the hair is yin.

What kind of hair shows the best digestive ability? Everyone has a different type of hair, even if they are blonde or brunette, European or Asian. They may have similar hair, but all will have a different condition of their hair. The five billion people in the world means that there are five billion different types of hair. It shows five billion different types of digestive ability. Hair can be thick or it can be thin. It can be smooth, or it can be dry and coarse. It can be strong, or it can be weak and brittle. Babies have fine, thin hair. Babies are very yang. So thin hair shows a very yang person. Thick hair shows a yin person. People who eat plenty of meat have thinner hair. Vegetable eating produces thick hair. This is the general principle.

Which do you think is better, weak, fragile hair or hair that is hard to break? The unbreakable hair is much better. Otherwise, when the handsome prince wanted to see the princess Rapunzel, he would not have been able to climb into her tower. He would have fallen down. What causes fragile hair? When hair is fragile, the elastic power is not there. Elasticity means that good-quality yin and good-quality yang are there. Then the hair can be springy. If not, then the hair will break easily. If we eat meat and sugar, our hair will become brittle and fragile.

When your hair falls out, that means that the intestinal villi are becoming inactive. Among animal foods, the food which causes the intestinal villi to become inactive are those which are most like baby food: dairy food and eggs. These foods make hair fall out. Complex carbohydrates make hair stronger and fuller. Too much protein from animal foods will cause hair to weaken and fall out. The eating of sugar will cause hair to become fragile. Many women today have weak hair. Their hair cannot hold their prince. Their hair cannot bind their sweetheart.

Both men and women may have hair with split ends. It is especially noticeable on men with long hair. What causes split ends? Yin or yang? The cause is yin. Split ends reflect the condition of the person's sexual organs. It shows the condition of the man's testis and the woman's ovaries. When these organs become yin, sexual power is decreased. The person who has split ends is very emotional and sensitive. He or she may feel insecure and confused, and have trouble making decisions.

Some people have bushy hair. Some people have straight hair. What causes this difference? Yang type of food, such as animal food, causes bushy or curly hair. Yin type food, especially vegetable food, causes straight hair. Various degrees of food are there, so various degrees of hair are there.

These principles can be applied not only to the hair on the top of the head, but also to the hair on the body. If body hair is silver colored or white, it shows that the person has eaten milk and dairy food. If the body hair is dark, especially along the spine, then the corresponding region inside the body is in trouble. That shows a yin condition. Often that occurs on the area of the back behind the lungs, and behind the stomach, kidneys, and intestines.

It is natural for a woman to have an abundance of hair on her head; much more so than a man. On the other hand, it is quite natural for a man to have much more body hair. If a man has plenty of hair on his head, it is a sign that he is less manly than he could be. A man's hair is naturally short. The shoulder is the borderline. If his hair is longer than that, it is a sign that he is too feminine. A woman's hair can go to the floor. Yin type of hair is naturally stimulated by eating yin type of food, such as grains, vegetables, and fruits, while yang type of hair is stimulated by eating animal food.

The color of the pubic hair should be the same as the rest of the hair on the head and body. But the direction of the growth of the hair is the opposite. The hair on the top of the head grows upward. The pubic hair grows downward. The hair on the top of the head should be thick. The pubic hair should be much less thick. The hair on the top of the head is the result of earth's force. The pubic hair is the result of heaven's force.

When there are some white or gray hairs on your head this is a strong yang sign. When we are children we have lighter hair. We are strongly yang then. If we eat too much salt, then our hair will become white or gray. In order to make white hair into dark hair, it is not difficult. You can eat more vegetables, more sea vegetables, and little salt. This transition will take a little time, but gradually your hair will become darker.

On the whole, hair shows a person's mental condition. Plenty of nice hair shows a pleasant and generous mentality. Bald, thin hair indicates a tight or stingy personality. The presence of dandruff reflects too much eating, especially protein such as fish, chicken, or other animal food. Moist hair is caused from taking in too much water. Oily hair is caused by eating plenty of oily, fatty food. Dry hair is caused by a lack of oil and water in the diet, or by too much saturated fat.

Hair Spirals

There are many spirals on the head. The top spiral on the head, the ears, the eyes, even the cheekbones are formed by a spiral. The spirals in the northern hemisphere turn in counterclockwise directions. Those in the southern hemisphere turn in a clockwise direction. You can test this in the bathtub or sink. When the water runs down the drain, it spirals counterclockwise in this hemisphere, but clockwise in the southern hemisphere.

The spiral on the head should not be exactly in the center of the head. Rather it should be a little bit behind the center of the head. The most balanced place for the spiral is in the middle of the head a little behind the exact center of the head. A person with a head spiral in this place is generally a balanced person—not too aggresive, not too negative—and has a tendency to see things in a fair or balanced way. Of these people, many are artistic.

A person who has a spiral on the right side of the head is generally a yang or active type of person. This kind of person is usually physically active and has a tendency to be socially active as well. On the other hand, a person with a hair spiral on the left side of the head is yin—more intellectual, mentally active, and artistic. This type of person will have a tendency toward engineering and calculations and an analytical way of thinking. This kind of person will love figures.

The distance from the top of the head to the center of the spiral indicates the latitude of the place of birth of the person. The force of heaven comes down directly to the north. But as our place of birth is not the direct north, the force comes down at an angle. If we were born at the exact north pole, the spiral would be close to the top of the head. But as none of us were born there, the spiral moves down the back of the head in proportion to the distance from the north pole and toward the equator.

What does it mean when a person has two head spirals? Is the person very clever, or very mad? The spiral is the entrance of heaven's force into the body. Ideally this channel should be the same one through which earth's force leaves the body. But in some cases this channel is not the same; instead two channels are formed. One channel serves heaven's force coming into the body; one channel serves earth's force leaving the body. The spiral that moves counterclockwise is the one receiving heaven's force. The spiral that goes clockwise is the one dispersing earth's force. This is the situation for people who are living in the northern hemisphere. If a man has two spirals his personality will evidence strong yin. If a woman has two spirals her personality will evidence strong yang. If a woman, while pregnant, eats strong yang and strong yin, and the the child is a girl, she may be born with two spirals. If the pregnant woman eats strong yin and the child is a boy, he may be born with two spirals.

Face

Of the three major systems: digestive, circulatory, and nervous, no one has all three in perfect condition. If someone has a strong digestive system, then probably either the circulatory or nervous system will be weaker. Because these three systems are complementary to each other, no one can possibly have all three in perfect condition. In the same respect a physically strong person may not be mentally agile. But a mentally agile person may not necessarily be physically strong. A person who is proficient in thinking in the dimension of time may not necessarily be proficient in dealing with space. If you have great love for your family and children, this does not necessarily mean that you have great love for your friends and society. The vertical and horizontal relations are opposite, so you may be stronger in the horizontal relations than in the vertical ones, or vice versa.

In all things we try to make balance. That is our major effort. We try to build up the weaker aspects of our thinking, our health, our physical condition, while maintaining the strength of our stronger points. If you have a great defect, a serious illness, then that is really an advantage. At the back side of this defect, you have something which is very strong to balance this weakness. Perhaps that is your mentality, or perhaps humility, or perhaps it is tendency toward hard work, or perhaps hard study, or perhaps love for other people. In any case you will have a superior point somewhere.

The condition of the nervous system and senses can be seen in the upper portion of the face, in the area of the forehead. This section ends in the tip of the nose. Thus, a long nose indicates that the nervous system is expanded. If the nose is long, a person may be brilliant, but his physical condition may be weak. The area between the nose and the mouth shows the condition of the reproductive organs. According to an Oriental proverb, if that area is large, it is an indication that the person is too sweet to the opposite sex. If the cheeks are contracted, it means that the circulatory system is strong. The lower part of the face, including the area around the mouth and chin, shows the condition of the digestive system. If the chin is expanded, it means that the digestive organs are well-developed. The person may be physically strong, but not necessarily brilliant.

The position of the features also reveals much about a person's constitution. If the face is expanded and the features are separated, the person has a yin constitution. But if the features are contracted and close together, the person has a yang constitution.

Forehead

The forehead shows your intellectuality. If the forehead is large, then your intellectual capacity is great. A narrow forehead shows a smaller capacity. The measurement is taken from the hairline to the top of the eyebrows. Everyone's forehead is different. No two foreheads are exactly alike. So everyone has a unique character, a unique mentality. Some people have a flat forehead. Some people have a forehead that sticks out. Why does this happen? What is the cause? When the forehead sticks out, it shows that the person can see clearly to his goal. He does not have to yield to anyone, but can straightly pursue his dream or purpose. This type of person is not wishy-washy.

If the center of the forehead is indented, it means that the region of the third eye is not coming out. It is better if this part of the forehead is slightly indented. The reason is that at the depth of the third eye lies the midbrain. The midbrain should be strongly yang. Thus it should be contracted. If this area juts out from the forehead in the form of a bump or some such protrusion, it indicates a tendency to be out of one's mind. It shows a lack of common sense. This kind of person has a tendency to be a something like a mad genius. Some people have a black mark, like a beauty mark, on the line from the scalp to the bridge of the nose in the center of the forehead. This is also not a good sign. In Oriental physiognomy a mark in this region is considered a sign of danger or misfortune.

When the forehead becomes oily or watery, it is an indication of excess in the bladder. This type of person will urinate frequently. Some people have blue vessels appearing on the sides of the forehead. The appearance of these vessels indicates that the opposite region—the intestines—are tight and contracted. Contraction of the intestines causes the vessels on the forehead to bulge. A person who has visible blue vessels on the forehead will also experience pain when pressure is applied to the hara region, showing that hardening of the arteries may be taking place. Hardening of the intestines is frequently a sign of high blood pressure.

If you have a beauty mark high on the temples near the scalp line, this is good. It is a sign of success. It also indicates that you will have good seniors or teachers who will help you to grow and develop. It shows a tendency toward achieving a high position.

Horizontal lines on the forehead are a sign of yin. They show a yin character. They indicate a tendency toward overdrinking. When you become older, you will develop these lines, especially when you shrink and become dehydrated. But also when you drink too much the area between the lines becomes swollen and wrinkles appear. There are two causes of horizontal lines; the first is yang , and the second yin.

Yin does not necessarily mean softness. Yin can also mean hardness. Take, for example, a bow and arrow. When you pull back the bow string, it is expanded—it is yin—but it is also becoming tight. The same thing happens in your body. When you eat ice cream, your intestines may expand, but the back side of the muscles along the spine become tight. When you apply pressure to that area it will be tight. That tightness is caused by too much yin. In this way yin causes hardness.

Also yin is low temperature. When coldness is applied to liquids they become solids. Ice is the typical example of this. Butter is another example. So, yin is not necessarily soft. It depends upon the condition. Yin creates a yang condition.

Rigidity can be caused by strong yin or by strong yang. Salt is one of the primary causes of rigidity. But it can also be caused by eating spices and drinking coffee and peppermint tea. The appearance of rigidity may be the same, but you must determine whether the cause is yin or yang.

We can also see what type of personality someone has by seeing the shape of the forehead. A person with a large forehead is usually an intellectual type. Someone with a sloping forehead is generally more active.

Eyebrows

Your eyebrows show your life history. The eyebrows begin at

the inner part of the face and develop outward toward the periphery. The inner third of the eyebrow shows your life as a baby. The middle third shows your life as an adult. The outer third of your eyebrow shows your life as an elderly person. If your eyebrow is long, that means you can live to an old age. If your eyebrow is short, that means you have less potential for longevity. If the hair on your eyebrow is thick or wide, and you have plenty of hair, and each one is long, that means you have the potential for a long, happy, and healthy life. If the hair on your eyebrows is thin, that means your native potential is less. If on the way from the beginning of the eyebrow to the end, there is a space, a break in the hair, that shows that at that time of your life you will experience some type of crisis, possibly a sickness or accident. It is similar to a break in the life line on the palm of the hand.

The eyebrows were formed during the period when we were in the mother's womb. After we are born we repeat this history in accordance with the pattern established in the uterus. Our whole life pattern is sct whcn we are in the womb.

To summarize, the length of the eyebrow indicates your potential for longevity. The thickness of eyebrow shows your vitality. If your eyebrows are thin, you have less vitality. But if your eyebrows are thick, you have a great deal of vitality. The width of the eyebrow indicates your capacity, the nature of your personality. A narrow eyebrow shows that you have a small capacity. A wide eyebrow shows that you have the capacity to understand and accept others.

The angle of the eyebrow shows what kind of food you have eaten. If the eyebrow slants up from the inside to the outside, it shows the past eating of animal food. If the eyebrow slants down from the inside toward the outside, it shows the past eating of vegetable food. The length of each hair shows your mental, spiritual understanding. If each hair is long, it shows that your mental, spiritual understanding is very great. If each hair is short, it shows that your spiritual, mental understanding is not as well-developed.

If the distance between the eyebrows is small, it is a sign of a yang person. This type of person is very tenacious. If the distance between the eyebrows is great, it is a sign of a yin person. This type of person has a tendency toward separation; including from parents, husband or wife, or children. A woman with eyebrows like this may experience the loss of her husband. In the Orient, this type of face is often referred to as a "widow's face."

Eyes

We can learn many things about a person's character by examining the shape and position of the eyes.

The left eye shows the influence of your father. The right eye shows the influence of your mother. If the left eye is smaller than the right, your father was more yang and active than your mother. If the right eye is smaller than the left, your mother was more yang and active than your father. When you use your eyes, you never use the two of them to the same degree. You use one eye more than the other. You use one eye to focus, and the other to create depth. If you see with only one eye you will not be able to see depth or dimension. Some people use their right eye to focus, while others use their left. There is a simple method to determine which eye you use to focus. Stretch your hand out in front of you. Align it with a spot on the far wall. Keep both eyes open and without moving your arm, close the left eye; then open it. Close the right eye; then open it. The eye that shows movement is the weaker eye. The eye that shows your hand in the same spot as when both eyes are open is the stronger eye.

In addition, you can see the influence of your grandparents in your eyes. The left eye indicates the father. The inner side of the eye shows the influence of your father's mother. The outer side of the left eye shows the influence of your father's father. In the same respect the right eye indicates the influence of your mother. The inner side of the right eye shows the influence of your mother's mother. The outer side of the the right eye shows the influence of your mother's father. That means that everyone's eyes differ in size and shape according to the influence of their parents and grandparents.

The size and shape of the eye as a whole indicates the influence of the parents. The degree of tightness at the ends of each eye indicates the influence of the grandparents. Tightness at the end of the eye indicates yang, while openness indicates yin. If the outer end of the right eye is tight, that means that the mother's father was a strong and active person. But if the inner end of the left eye is open, that means that the father's mother had a weaker condition.

If the eyes slant upward from the inner part of the face to the outer part, that person is yang. If the eyes slant downward from the inner to the outer end, that person is yin. The best condition is for the eyes to lie straight across the face. If the eyebrows slope downward, while the eyes themselves slant upward, what does this mean? The eyebrows are yin, but the eyes are yang. This indicates that the person has eaten vegetable food, but yang vegetable food, especially carrots, burdock root, and salty pickled vegetables. The opposite condition is where the eyebrows are sloping upward while the eyes themselves are slanting downward. This indicates that the person has eaten a lot of animal food, yet that person is yin.

If there is a straight line drawn down the center of the face, no one will have an exactly symmetrical formation on both sides. This occurs because the influence received from the mother is different from that received from the father. This variation in influence will cause one side to be yang and the other side to be yin. One side will be contracted, while the other side will be expanded. So if you take a picture of one side of a person's face and put it next to a picture of the other side, both sides will appear very different. Try this with a photograph and you will be surprised.

Now let us look at the eye itself. The inner half of the eye is yang, while the outer half is yin. The lower half of the eye is also yang, while the upper half is yin. Each section of the eye corresponds to one of the organs of the body. These correspondences are presented in the diagram.

The Eye with Correspondences

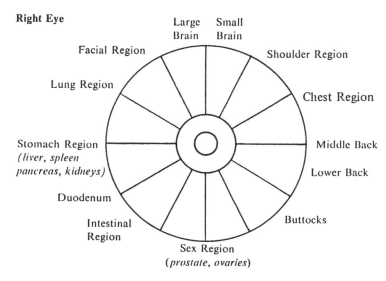

Right Eye

Large Brain — Small Brain

Facial Region

Shoulder Region

Lung Region

Chest Region

Stomach Region
*(liver, spleen
pancreas, kidneys)*

Middle Back

Lower Back

Duodenum

Intestinal
Region

Buttocks

Sex Region
(*prostate, ovaries*)

The appearance of blood vessels within the white portion of the eye indicates a weakness in the organ that corresponds to the section in which the blood vessel lies. If there is a blood vessel in the area of the cerebrum, in the upper region of the eye, that means the cerebrum is expanded. When we were babies, none of us had blood vessels in our eyeball. As we become older, many blood vessels appear, especially when we are tired. That means that your blood vessels and your circulation have become expanded. The blood vessels are moving toward the periphery, instead of being toward the inside where they were when you were a baby.

When your eyes are bloodshot, and there is a small dot at the end of the vessel, the color of the dot is important. If the dot is red, it indicates a blood clot in the organ corresponding to the area of the eye. If the dot is dark, that indicates stone formation. Often the stomach, kidney, or spleen region will have an indication of stone formation. Or around there mucus splotches, like tofu or cheese, will appear, showing that within that part of the body, fat deposits are developing. Cysts may also be forming. This marking frequently appears in the middle region of the eye, the region that shows the condition of the breasts, indicating that fat and mucus are accumulating there, possibly in the form of cysts. If there is a greenish shade around that mucus deposit, it is a sign that cancer may be developing.

Blood vessels or dots frequently appear in the lower region of the eye that corresponds to the kidneys and sex organs. If the dot or vessel is white, it indicates that a cyst is forming, such as an ovarian cyst or dermoid tumor. If it is dark, it shows the formation of a kidney stone. If it is yellow, it indicates that deposits of fat are accumulating. If it is red, it indicates that a blood clot may be developing.

The method of detecting conditions by examining the iris is called iridology. But in order to detect accurately, we need to use a magnifying glass. In some cases we can plainly see the indications of weakness in the organs. But in many cases, the indications are so slight that we need to have them magnified in order to see them properly.

If along the area of the pancreas and intestinal region, especially near the edge of the white of the eye, you see a white, transparent mucus deposit, that indicates that you have been eating too much dairy food and sugar. If along the edge of the rest of the white of the eye you see a yellowish colored deposit, that indicates that you have too much fatty acid in your body, probably caused by eating too much dairy food and eggs.

The white of the eye should generally be clear and free of markings. If there is any red color, that indicates that the bloodstream, or circulatory system, is in trouble. If there is a yellow color, that indicates that the middle digestive organs are in trouble. If there is a dark color (you may say black), that indicates that the kidneys and excretory system are in trouble. If there is a blue or purple color that indicates that the spleen and nervous system are in trouble. If there is a green color, that is an indication of cancer.

Ears

The three areas can be viewed on the ear. The innermost ridge of the ear shows the condition of the digestive and respiratory systems. The middle ridge shows the condition of the nervous system, and the outermost ridge of the ear shows the condition of the circulatory and excretory systems.

Ideally, the ear should be situated on the head so that the bottom of the lobe is directly in line with the mouth, while the top of the ear is directly in line with the eyes. Ears that rise above the eye line are yang. Ears that go below the mouth line are yin. The development of the earlobe indicates the development of the brain. Traditionally, it was considered a good sign to have long earlobes. They were thought to be a sign of wisdom and spiritual insight. Perhaps you have seen your grandparents, or people of that generation. Many of them have well-developed earlobes.

A large ear is a good sign. If the ear is large, that indicates that inside the organs are properly contracted and vitally active. If your ear is large from top to bottom, that means that you can hear from both heaven and earth. So, your judgment is clear. If your ear is flat against your head, you can hear from the front, from the side, from the back. So, again, the scope of your reception of vibrations is large.

The ideal ear has the upper and lower portions both developed. Overconsumption of protein, even from animal sources, will cause the upper portion of the ear to be well-developed, and the lower portion to be underdeveloped. An excess of carbohydrate, especially simple sugar, potatoes, and refined flour, causes the middle portion to be well-developed, but the upper portion and the earlobe are underdeveloped. The earlobe is the coldest place on the body. Often when a person burns his finger, he will unconsciously tug on his earlobe for relief. Minerals gather in the earlobe and cause it to develop. Ears that lie close to the head are yang. Ears that stick out are yin. Ears may jut from the head up to an angle of thirty degrees. After that they are too yin.

The development of the ear is not hereditary at all. The size and shape of the ear indicates the food which the baby's mother was eating. After the baby is born, up to about ten or twelve years old, gradual changes can be affected, but we cannot change the structure of the ear completely. The ear shows the constitution of the mother, especially during the first three months of pregnancy when the ears were developing. So, we cannot change them much. But do not be disappointed. We may not be able to change the structure of the ears, but we can change their nature. That we can do with macrobiotics.

Nose

The nose shows the condition of the heart and lungs. The tip of the nose indicates the heart. If the tip of the nose is sharp and pointed, then the heart is very yang. If the tip of the nose is red and swollen, then the heart is expanded. This condition arises among people who drink a lot of alcohol. A split at the tip of the nose shows that the valves of the heart are not closing properly. The nostrils show the condition of the lungs. Well-developed nostrils show well-developed and strong lungs. Nostrils that are flaccid and underdeveloped reveal potential weakness in the lungs. The shape of the nose also shows a person's constitution. A long, drooping nose indicates a yin constitution. A short, pug nose indicates a yang constitution, and a straight, well-proportioned nose indicates a well-balanced constitution.

Mouth

The upper lip shows the condition of the stomach. The lower lip shows the condition of the large and small intestines. If either or both of the lips are swollen, this indicates that there is too much excess in these organs. The person most likely suffers from stomach trouble, or from chronic constipation or other digestive disorders. The well-proportioned mouth should extend to the outer limits of the nostrils, and no farther. This is a sign of good-quality yang. A mouth that extends beyond the nostrils indicates that the digestive system is natively yin with the potential for weakness and digestive troubles. Vertical lines on the lower lip often indicate diarrhea, while a swollen lower lip may be a sign of chronic constipation.

Teeth

We have thirty-two teeth: sixteen upper and sixteen lower. Four are used for cutting, two are used for tearing (the canine teeth), and ten are used for grinding. In each quadrant of the mouth this means that there are two cutting teeth, one tearing tooth, and five grinding teeth, in a ratio of 2:1:5=8. From this proportion we can see that our diet should consist of two parts vegetables, one part animal food (primarily white-meat fish in temperate zones), and five parts grains and beans. This proportion also reflects our biological history since organisms first appeared upon this earth 3.2 billion years ago.

Because of our biological heritage, which we see reflected in the structure of the teeth, the ideal human diet consists of seven parts vegetable food to one part animal food. In a temperate climate, low-fat, white-meat fish is the most appropriate form of animal food. When you travel from a cold climate where you are eating a large percentage of grain, to a warm climate, should you eat more vegetables and less grains? No. The proportion of grains and vegetables should remain the same. What may change is the type of grains and vegetables you use. In a cold climate eat more yang grains and vegetables; in a warm climate eat more yin grains and vegetables. In a cold climate eat short-grain rice; in a warm climate you can eat more long-grain rice. The proportion of foods we should eat is already determined for us by the kind of teeth we are born with.

If a person's teeth jut out, for example, in buck teeth, that is a sign of yin. This formation is caused by eating too much fruit. Teeth that go inward are a sign of yang, and result from too much salt, fish, and meat.

If you have spaces between your teeth, especially between the two front teeth, it is a sign that you are too yin. It is a sign of separation, a sign that you may not be able to see your parents at the time of their death. Separation between the teeth is caused by a jaw that is overly big and expanded. If you are taking too much liquid, fruit juice, and salad, and too many sweets, your teeth may start to separate.

When you close your teeth, they should meet in an orderly and balanced manner. Overbite, where the upper teeth jut out over the lower teeth, is yin. On the other hand, when the lower teeth jut out over the upper teeth, the cause is too much yang.

Tongue

The shape of the tongue is an indication of the condition of a person's constitution. Grain and vegetable eating produces a tongue that is short and thick, with a rounded end. A diet high in animal food produces a tongue that is long and pointed. If the tongue has an indentation at the tip, the cause is strong yin. This condition is similar to having a split in the tip of the nose, which is also caused by eating strong yin. In order to taste food, but more importantly, in order to speak well, the tongue should be wide and round. That is the best shape for good speaking. The shape of the tongue influences not only speech, but the choice of words.

The tongue is the end of the digestive vessel, and it shows the condition of the internal digestive organs. If the tongue is coated with a yellow color, the liver, gallbladder, and pancreas are in trouble. If the tongue is bright red, the stomach or intestines are suffering from ulcers and possibly cancer. If the tongue is coated with white, there is an excess of mucus in the stomach. When you have a high fever, the color of your tongue will become white. Mucus is trying to be discharged, that is why you are having a high fever.

Facial Lines

Everyone has a variety of lines on the face. These lines tell us about the condition of the internal organs and about how a person has been eating and drinking. The area on the bridge of the nose indicates the condition of the liver, pancreas, and spleen. Vertical lines on the bridge of the nose are caused by accumulation of mucus and fat in the liver, and expansion or hardening of the liver. The deeper and longer the wrinkles are, the worse the condition is. There may be only one line, or several. If only one or two, the liver is harder and more rigid, with stagnation in its functions. These wrinkles show that hard fats are also accumulating in the gallbladder, and may indicate gallstones. Vertical lines in the region of the face that corresponds to the liver show a mental tendency toward upset, short temper, and anger.

One horizontal line on the bridge of the nose indicates hardening and tightness in the pancreas, caused by eating too much animal food, especially chicken, cheese, eggs, and shellfish. It frequently indicates hypoglycemia, or chronic low blood sugar, together with fatigue, a craving for sweets, and the tendency toward depression or anxiety.

A vertical line in the space between the nose and the upper lip is a sign of too much yang in the sexual organs. If a woman has this line she will probably suffer from pain during menstruation. If the area between the nose and the upper lip is swollen and rounded, this indicates that there is too much mucus in the stomach, spleen, and pancreas.

Hands

The thumb is the center of the hand; it can fit into a tightly clenched fist. Therefore it is very strong; it is the most yang part of the hand. A monkey has a thumb, but he cannot move his thumb. It is not flexible like the human thumb. The monkey's thumb can only move in the same direction as the other fingers.

Because of this, the monkey's hand is not as dexterous as the human hand. A highly mobile thumb is unique to the human hand. The monkey's thumb developed by eating fruit. The human thumb developed as a result of eating cereal grains. The eating of fruit will cause the human thumb to become less flexible. The disease associated with the loss of finger and thumb flexibility is called arthritis.

Recently many babies are being born with webbing between their fingers. This is a characteristic of frogs and ducks, but is not a normal condition for humans. When a pregnant mother drinks orange juice, soft drinks, and eats strong yin foods, these cancel out the contracting effect of minerals and other yang factors. This can cause a baby to be born with webbing between the fingers. This means that the fingers have not sufficiently contracted. They have not sufficiently separated one from another. Usually when a baby is born with a large amount of webbing, the doctor will operate to remove the excess skin. Thus the hand will appear normal, but the person will still have an overly yin condition.

Your fingers should be flexible. Your fingers should be able to bend backward at least ninety degrees. The degree of flexibility evidenced by your fingers shows the flexibility of your brain. If your fingers are not flexible, then your thinking will tend to be rigid, stubborn, and one-sided.

When you make a fist, the spaces between your knuckles should be well-indented. If they are not, this shows that you have many fatty deposits in your spleen, liver, and pancreas. These deposits develop from eating too much sugar and gourmet food. This also indicates hardening of the arteries and joints. This condition can easily be corrected with a good macrobiotic diet.

When you hold your hand straight upright, it is better if there are no spaces between your fingers. If your hand does have spaces, then you will not be able to hold water in your hand, nor money, or so people say. Spaces between the fingers correspond to spaces between the teeth. When you have spaces between your fingers, it means that you are a yin type of person, that you do not have togetherness. You may be lazy and may have difficulties living with other people. You may also have a difficult time with discipline. That is why, as a result, this kind of person cannot hold money. So this kind of person should eat well to compensate for this yin type of constitution. Then he can hold money.

The temperature of the hand when you touch it should not be warm, nor should it be cold. Rather it should be slightly cool. Also, the hand should not be moist. It should be dry. A person with a moist hand is taking too much liquid, including too much fruit juice. Moist hands indicate that the heart and kidneys are overworking. This type of person is a slow thinking person; his mechanical ability will also be somewhat slow. Generally speaking, this is a yin condition.

The Life Line

The life line shows the condition of the respiratory and digestive systems. It begins over the thumb and circles around the base of

The Hand with Important Lines

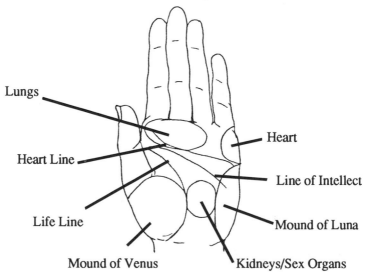

Lungs

Heart

Heart Line

Life Line

Line of Intellect

Mound of Luna

Mound of Venus

Kidneys/Sex Organs

the thumb toward the wrist. Actually the life line should end at the place where you take the pulse. The life line is formed during pregnancy, and during our life we repeat that period. The life line should be long, clear, and deep. That means that the digestive vessels are strong. It indicates that the mother was healthy and ate well. Thus, the person has the potential to be strong and healthy.

If the life line is dim, or weak, that means that your life pattern is weak. And if you have minute lines crossing the life line on the perpendicular, it indicates that you will suffer from many minor conditions. If the life line is broken, it means that at the period in your life that corresponds to the area of the break, you will have some trouble, perhaps sickness or an accident.

If the life line becomes dim during its course around the base of the thumb, it indicates that a chronic illness will occur during that period of life. A broken line indicates a sudden occurrence, while a fading line indicates a chronic illness. If an island appears on the life line, that means that some sickness or difficulty will arise at that time. If the life line is doubled, it is not necessarily bad, but indicates that your life pattern is complicated. So instead of having one wife, you may have two. Instead of one job, you may have two. When a person has a double life line, the cause is a yin one. The little parallel lines on the base of the thumb are caused by yang.

The Line of Intellect

The line of intellect shows the condition of the nervous system. If it is long, the person will be a more yin type. If the line of intellect is short, the person is yang. Again, this line should be deep and clear. If this line if fragile, it is an indication of potential weakness in the nervous system. The person may be overly sensitive or nervous.

When the line of intellect droops down toward the base of the palm, it indicates a yin type of person. When the line of intellect goes up toward the fingers, it indicates that the person is yang. The life line should be long, but the line of intellect does not necessarily have to be long. During the formation of the fetus, the spiral of the nervous system is tighter, thus the line of the nervous system should be yang. The spiral of the digestive system is more extended, thus the line of the digestive system can be longer, more yin. The length of the line of intellect is not as important as its being clear and deeply etched across the hand. If this condition exists, then the nervous system is strong.

The line of intellect begins just above the thumb and continues across the hand toward the outer edge. The far end of the line of intellect shows the condition of the brain. The beginning of the line of intellect shows the condition of the base of the spine. The middle part of the line of intellect shows the condition of the spine as it rises from the base to the brain.

At the center of the line of intellect is a point called the heart of the hand. The heart of the hand usually coincides with the point where the line of intellect crosses the fate line, or the line that rises from the wrist to the center of the middle finger in the center of the palm. The fate line, when it is long and deep, is an indication that the person is a hard worker. Another important line is the line of success. It rises from the wrist and goes toward the little finger. This line may be short when a person is young, but the more hardworking a person is, the longer the line of success may become.

The Heart Line

The heart line begins at the outer edge of the hand directly beneath the little finger and proceeds across the palm. It indicates the condition of the circulatory system. This line, again, should be deeply etched and clear and bold. If the heart line ends toward the index finger, it is an indication that the circulatory system is yin. But if the heart line is short, it is an indication that the circulatory system is very yang.

The point at which the heart line crosses an imaginary line that runs down the center of the middle finger, shows the condition of the kidneys. If you press the part of the palm just underneath the little finger, and detect hardness there, or if the person feels soreness, it shows the potential for heart trouble. If you press in a similar manner under the middle finger and there is hardness or soreness, then the kidneys are in trouble. When the heart line joins with the line of intellect, this is a strong yang sign. A person with this formation is a very yang person.

The Mounds

The mounds, or raised areas on the inside of the palm, also reveal the internal condition. These are shown in the diagram above. The mound of Venus indicates the condition of the large intestine. When you push there and you feel soreness, or if the mound has a blue or purple color, then you know the large intestine is in trouble. The mound of Luna indicates the condition of the small intestine. Between the mound of Venus and the mound of Luna lies the area which indicates the condition of the kidneys and sex organs. This area is not exactly in the center of the palm, but is a little below center. If you feel pain when this area is pressed, then your kidneys or sex organs are in trouble.

The center of the palm indicates the condition of the nervous system, the brain, and especially the midbrain. The mound just under the little finger indicates the condition of the heart. The mound under the index finger indicates the condition of the lungs. The area of the lung can be extended to cover the mounds of the other fingers. The other organs such as the liver, stomach, and spleen do not appear so much in the palm of the hand. Their condition can more easily be read by the appearance of the feet.

Other Lines

A line of health, which runs from the little finger down toward the wrist, is a good sign. If you have this line, it is very good. Those lines which are usually referred to as the marriage lines can be found on the outside edge of the palm just below the little finger. They run parallel to the heart line and are usually short. Usually people say that you can tell how many marriages you will have by the number of lines you have. But this is not the case. Nor is it correct to assume that the number of little lines that cross the marriage lines perpendicularly indicate the number of children you will have. More than two marriage lines is not a good sign. These lines indicate the regularity or irregularity of the heartbeat. If there are too many lines, that indicates that the beating of the heart is irregular. Ideally, there should only be one marriage line. This would indicate regular heart beating.

Fingers

The reverse side of the hand is not so interesting as the palm. But there is something to be understood by examining the size and shape of the fingers. First of all, you should see if the fingers are straight. Straight fingers indicate an orderly person. But many people have curved fingers.

If the fingers are curved toward the thumb, this is a yang sign.

If the fingers are curved toward the little finger, this is a yin sign.

If the fingers are curved toward the middle finger, this shows that both strong yin and strong yang are there. While the person was growing, he took plenty of meat and sugar.

The thumb is the finger of the parents. The index finger is the finger of those who are older, such as older brothers or sisters. The middle finger is the finger of yourself. The ring finger is the finger of your brothers and sisters. The little finger is the finger of your children. If your other fingers are leaning toward the thumb, that means that you are depending upon your parents. If your fingers lean toward the ring or little fingers, then you will have a tendency toward the younger generation, and these people are going to take care of you in the future. You will be under their protection, economically and socially. If the finger of the younger brothers and sisters leans toward the finger of yourself, then that means you will be taking care of them.

The relationship between the index finger and the ring finger is important. Ideally they should be of the same length. If the index finger is shorter than the ring finger, that indicates that your circulatory system is natively weak. If the index finger is longer than the ring finger, that indicates that your large intestine is natively weak.

Nails

The white moons at the base of the nails show the speed of your growth, which is yin. It is interesting to notice that children usually have large moons because they are growing very fast. But as they grow older, the size of their moons becomes smaller because the speed of growth becomes less. Then finally the moons should disappear altogether, especially by the time you are thirty-five years old. Except for the thumb, none of the other fingers should show moons by the time you are thirty-five years old.

Here and there white dots may appear on your nails. These dots indicate excessive intake of simple sugars, including those in refined sugar, fruit, and honey. They show yin being discharged through the nails. Suppose it takes six to seven months for the nail to grow from the cuticle out to the edge. And if you are older than thirty years it will probably take nine months for this growth to occur. If it takes your nail six months to grow out, then you can plot the time of your excessive intake by the exact position of the white spots.

If there is an indentation in the center of your nail, or if the nail feels mushy or soft in the center, that is an indication of worms. If there are vertical lines or ridges on your nails, it is a sign of too much yang, especially too much salt. To correct this imbalance, eat a little bit more oil in your diet. If you look at your nail from the side, and it appears to be wavy, it shows that you have had several changes in your diet. The places where the nail is mounded indicate a yin diet. The places where the nail is depressed indicate a yang diet. This kind of wavy nail condition is sometimes seen in people who travel a lot, who change from a warm climate to a cold climate and then back again to a warm climate.

Seeing the Mind and Emotions

Each of the meridians serves as a channel for waves of energy that carry thoughts, emotions, and consciousness. Each of the body's cells receives energy from the meridians, and acts as a center of consciousness. The meridians begin and end in the chakras and the fingers and toes. The correspondences between the meridians, fingers and toes, and characteristics of consciousness are presented in the tables below.

Correlation between Meridians and Aspects of Consciousness (Hand)

Meridian	Finger	Aspect of Consciousness	Function
Lung	Thumb	Intellect	Activating
Large Intestine	Index	Social awareness	Stabilizing
Heart Governor	Middle	Emotion, intellect, Social awarness	Activating
Triple Heater	Ring	Emotion, intellect social awareness	Stabilizing
Heart	Pinky (inside)	Emotion, intellect	Activating
Small Intestine	Pinky (outside)	Emotion, intellect	Stabilizing

The condition of the fingers and toes reveals the condition of these mental and emotional functions. If the fingers and toes are curved or twisted, rather than straight and orderly, if they are distorted because of arthritis, or if the condition of the nails is irregular, the corresponding mental and emotional functions are also being affected. Functional changes, including swelling, the presence of calluses, discoloration, and skin markings reveal dishar

Correlation between Meridians and Aspects
of Consciousness (Foot)

Meridian	Toe or Part of Foot	Aspect of Consciousness	Function
Spleen	First (outside)	Expression, emotion, intellect, social awareness, sex	Activating
Liver	First (inside)	Intellect, social awareness, sex	Activating
Stomach	Second and Third	Intellect	Stabilizing
Gallbladder	Fourth	Intellect, sex	Stabilizing
Bladder	Fifth	Expression, emotion, intellect, social awareness, sex	Stabilizing
Kidney	Bottom of Foot	Expression, emotion, social awareness, sex	Activating

mony in the flow of energy to the particular meridian, and in the condition of the organ and the mental and emotional conditions that correspond to it.

The mental and emotional condition can also be seen by looking at other parts of the meridian. Imbalances in daily diet and way of life cause the normally clean and clear skin color along the meridians to change, indicating imbalance in the related organs, glands, systems, and energy flow. These changes arise most often on the periphery of the meridian—at the arms and hands, the legs and feet, and on the face. Skin markings such as pimples, moles, and calluses that appear along a meridian indicate imbalances in the flow of mental and emotional energy, as do other abnormal features such as discoloration and excessive body hair. Often, the meridian may be seen to be either sunken or swollen in certain areas along its entire surface course. The swollen condition reflects an excess of energy and the sunken condition a deficiency.

Dimensions of Diagnosis

In our studies of diagnosis, I have presented many types of information; but many people have not questioned this information. For example, we understand that the area around the mouth shows the condition of the sex organs. This you may already know very well, and you may have confirmed that through practical experience; but did you ask why?

This is actually not so difficult to answer: as you know, the mouth itself lies at the end of the long digestive tract. What lies at the other end of that tract? The anus; so around the mouth and around the anus, there is a strong correlation. If your mouth is loose and swollen, then you know that you anus is also loose; if your lips are firm and tightly closed, then your anus is contracted and tight. The sex organs lie near the anus; therefore their condition appears around the mouth.

There are so many things like this that we need to question; for example, why do the lungs appear on the cheeks? Or, why does the heart correlate to the tip of the nose? As I explain in *How to See Your Health: The Book of Oriental Diagnosis* (Tokyo and New York: Japan Publications, Inc., 1980), the nose itself is formed as an extension of the nervous system. So a long, drooping nose indicates that the nervous system is expanded, while a short, tight nose shows a yang, practical-minded nervous system. But why does the heart appear there? How does that correlate to the nervous system?

When you begin to answer these questions for yourself, then your diagnosis will start to have much more depth; then you will be able to discover many things on your own, and not be limited to things that others have taught you.

Constitution at Conception

Suppose you want to know about a person's early embryonic condition; if possible, you would like to know what his condition was like when his parents' reproductive cells first combined. So somewhere on the face, while you are talking with him, you want to see where that original egg and sperm appear.

The father's sperm appears in the nose, while the mother's egg appears in the mouth. If the person's mouth is large, the egg was large and fragile. If the mouth is small and tight, the egg was dense and compact, more sturdy. The shape of the nose also shows the general shape of the person's father's sperm at the time of conception, with the tip and nostrils showing the sperm's head, and the bridge and length of the nose showing the sperm's tail. Of course, this may be somewhat influenced during the person's growing period; for example, if he ate plenty of fruit while he was growing up, then his nose will become longer; but the original generally remains.

Reproductive Organs

The condition of the uterus and ovaries appears around the mouth. But suppose you need to have an enlarged view, so you can see in greater detail. For that, you can use the whole face: the mouth represents the vagina, going up toward the uterus, represented by the nose. The ovaries appear in the eyes; if the right eye is bloodshot, then you know that there is some inflammation in the right ovary. If woman's nasal cavity is clogged with mucus, then you know that there is mucus building up in the uterus.

The male sex organs also are represented in the face: you can see the constitution and condition of the penis in the nose; the testicles are represented by the eyes, and the condition of the prostate appears in the area between the eyebrows.

Lungs

Suppose you are seeing someone who has a tumor beginning to grow in their lung; this you may be able to determine from techniques you already know, such as the general appearance of the cheeks, which may be slightly green, or you may see a green color around the base of the thumb when you press points on the lung meridian. Now, you want to know, exactly where in that lung is that tumor appearing?

Again, we need to see an enlarged view of the lungs, using the whole face. First, we need to see the area where our breath enters, or the bronchi; where does our breath enter on the face? Through the nasal passages; so, you can see the condition of the bronchi in detail around the outside of the bridge of the nose. Then, the lungs themselves appear as an inverted, or upside-down image on the face as a whole. The left side of the face corresponds to the left lung; the right side, to the right lung. If you see a pimple appearing on the lower part of the left side of the face, that indicates an accumulation of excess fats or sugar in the upper part of the left lung: a pimple in the upper part of the face would indicate trouble in the lower part of the corresponding lung. A black mark in the middle region of the face would show an accumulation of stagnated blood and minerals, like a carbon deposit, in the middle region of the lung.

Heart

As we saw above, the general condition of the heart appears in the tip of the nose, where you can detect whether the heart is swollen, hard, soft, whether the two chambers of the heart are coordinating well or poorly, and various other general conditions. But for a specific, enlarged view, we can again use the face as a whole.

In the diagram, you can see several important areas of the heart: A and B represent the right and left chambers of the heart; C and D represent the right atrium and ventricle, or upper and lower region, and E and F represent the left atrium and ventricle; X and Y and X 1 and Y 1 represent the flow of blood from the body to the heart and heart to the lung on the right side, and from the lung to the heart and the heart back to the body on the left side. N and N 1 represent the valves between the atrium and ventricle of each chamber.

The Heart (Schematic)

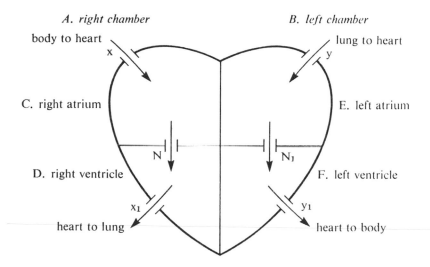

A. right chamber   *B. left chamber*

body to heart   lung to heart

x   y

C. right atrium   E. left atrium

N   N₁

D. right ventricle   F. left ventricle

x₁   y₁

heart to lung   heart to body

A and B appear in the right and left sides of the face, in general. Where can you see the borderline between areas C and D and E and F? To figure this out, you need to first see the actual flow of blood. The incoming flow of blood from the body to heart and lung to heart, areas X and X 1, corresponds to the canals from the outer ear in toward the inner ear; if you see the size of the ear's opening, that represents the size of that opening to the heart; if mucus or liquid is accumulating there, that shows similar accumulations in that area of the heart. Then, the flow of blood from heart to lung and from heart to body, areas Y and Y 1, appear in the nasal canal passages. Incidentally, the X and X 1 areas are much more commonly troubled than the Y and Y 1 areas.

Then, where can we see the actual valves, shown as N and N 1? Their condition is shown in the eyes. For good, strong heart functions those valves should be tight and strong; if the eyes become weak or watery, with frequent blinking, then those valves are becoming weak and watery. If the eyes are swollen or red,

Diagnosis of the Heart in the Face

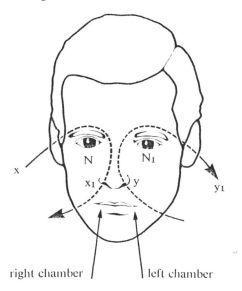

right chamber | left chamber

then some swelling or light inflammation is occurring in the corresponding valves. If the eyes are discharging mucus, then mucus is also accumulating around the valves.

The general condition of areas A and B, the right and left chambers, also appears in the mouth: for example, if the right side of the mouth is swollen or loose, this reflects a similar condition in the right chamber. If the mouth as a whole is becoming overexpanded and loose, the heart is overall becoming loose and weak. You can also see the heart's activity by the mouth's activity; a talkative person is usually associated with an expanded, overactive heart. You can also judge the overall coordination of the two chambers by seeing how well the two sides of the mouth coordinate when the person is speaking, and by the degree of balance or imbalance of the two sides while the mouth is at rest.

You can further refine this view by refining the exact correspondences; for example, if you see fatty accumulations or pimples appearing in one cheek, that indicates a corresponding accumulation in the wall of the chamber on that side of the body. You can further check for discoloration, pimples, blemishes and other indications in those areas. Then, if the face as a whole is bright red or pink, the heart is overworking, usually from too much liquid. If you can see individual capillaries appearing, then the heart is expanded and the person has the tendency toward high blood pressure. If the face becomes pale, then the heart has become either very tight or very weak, in either case resulting in an underactive condition.

Diagnosis of the Heart in the Hands.

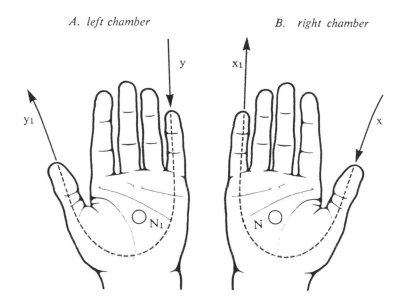

A. *left chamber*   B.   *right chamber*

The condition of the heart can also be seen in the hands. The right chamber, area A appears in the right hand; the left chamber, or region B, appears in the left hand. The hands also mirror the flow of blood in the heart.

In which region of the hand do you see generally more red color? Around the periphery; that is, along the thumb and little finger area. The flow of blood through both chambers is represented by the arrows in the diagram, beginning at the tip of the little finger, circulating along the periphery of the hand, and continuing out the thumb. Then, you can correlate any symptom appearing along that path to the corresponding region of blood flow in the heart. For example, you may see a chipped or discolored nail on the thumb or little finger; or if you see a dark discoloration in the fleshy part of the base of the thumb, which indicates stagnation in the large intestine, that is also indicating some stagnation in the upper middle area of blood flow within the heart.

The condition of the two central valves, marked N and N 1, appears directly in the center of each palm; if that area is swollen or expanded, or discolored, or if the person experiences pain when you push on that place, these all indicate related troubles with the corresponding valve, such as looseness, weakness, accumulation of fats or liquid, hardness, and so forth. If you have the so-called line of success, which runs straight down through this area, this indicates that your valves N and N 1 are constitutionally strong.

The strength of the grip of each hand shows generally the strength of each chamber; a comparison of the two hands will show generally how well the two chambers of the heart are coordinating, and therefore, how efficient the heart's activity is. For example, in structural terms, if the size, shape, major lines on the palms, and other general features of the hands are different, then the two chambers are different. Also in terms of activity, when a person uses his hands, you can check whether the two hands are working together well or not: this also shows how well the two heart chambers are working together. If the two chambers are not working together in a smoothly coordinated, harmonious way, then some irregularity of heartbeat will result. This in turn will produce a tendency of the emotions and of the overall character to fluctuate between extremes, rather than to be consistent, steady, and dependable.

Such an imbalanced right-left condition will also reflect in all the various paired organs, such as the two kidneys, the two lungs, the liver and spleen, or the two halves of the brain and two sides of the face. You can also compare the pulses on the right and left wrists. If the right and left pulses are not exactly coordinated, which you can detect by taking pulses on both hands simultaneously, this would indicate some serious imbalance between the right and left sides of the heart and body as a whole.

You can go on to see all the organs with this in-depth view, to deepen your understanding of diagnosis; also, remember that everything is different, nothing is identical to anything else. For example, we usually look from the front, but in the case of, for example, the kidneys, if you want to see an enlarged view, it is better to see from the side. Also sometimes you have a clearer view if you see an upside-down image of that organ, as we saw with the lungs. In other words, you cannot develop this kind of diagnosis mechanically: you must really reflect on those organs, and really use your intuition.

Until now, I have presented only the basics of Oriental diagnosis; and that is enough for practical, simple purposes. But in order to guide people, to become a healer and teacher of the view of life, and to develop your understanding of the universe, you should not rest there but go far, far beyond those basic studies.

Diagnosis of Mental/Psychological Tendencies

As we stand upon the earth, we are receiving earth's force and heaven's force, creating one unified vertical channel, or central axis. When we deviate from this axis, entering a horizontal dimension, we call that movement in terms of the body, and mind or thought in terms of the head. This deviation may be very horizontal, or mildly horizontal and mildly vertical, with many different variations; that range of different motions in the horizontal dimensions we call our relative judgment and actions.

If we are healthy and energetic, we are like a spinning, charged top: we always spontaneously right ourselves and return to that central, vertical axis. This return to the vertical dimension, or cessation of relative thought and action, we call instinct in terms of the body, and intuition in terms of the head; together, our intuitive instinct and instinctive intuition comprise our absolute judgment.

In order to see a person's mind, in other words, his relative judgment, character, and personality, we can look at the horizontal structure of his body. As an example, we can distinguish seven horizontal divisions of the face.

1. The jaw shows mental structure; a big jaw shows a person has a big mind, encompassing large dimensions, while a small jaw indicates a smaller mind. Also, there are generally three types of jaws: a square jaw, indicating a yang, practical mind; a round jaw, showing a balanced, harmonious mind; and a triangular jaw, which corresponds to a more intellectual mind.

2. The mouth shows mental discipline; a person with a tight, small mouth has strong self-discipline; a loose, bigger, or more open mouth shows that that person is also loose in his mental discipline or self-control. You may have noticed that when you want to do something requiring intense energy, like carrying a heavy object or thinking hard, you must close your mouth; if you open your mouth, you lose your body's power and your mind's power. (That is one reason why it is wise not to talk or eat too much!) What does a large mouth mean, in terms of embryology? It means that your mother did not exercise strong self-control in her eating when she was pregnant, and ate large quantities of extreme foods; then that trait is carried over to you. Also, if your lungs and sinus cavities become clogged, you cannot breathe freely through your nose, so you may leave your mouth hanging open; this again shows poor mental concentration or control.

3. The nose and nostrils show mental vitality or strength, or you might say whether or not the person has guts. Smaller nostrils show that the person's mental strength and conviction are not so strong; he has no guts; larger nostrils show that person has guts and mental vitality.

4. The ears show mental capacity: a person with larger ears or ears that lie flatter against the head can embrace various different opinions, while a person with smaller ears or ears

that stick out is mentally narrow, and has the tendency to alienate people with opinions foreign to his or her own.

5. The eyes show mental alertness and clarity. In terms of condition, eyes that are bloodshot, cloudy and dull show mental dullness, while sharp, clear eyes show an alert, penetrating mentality. Less blinking shows mental clarity, although if an adult does not blink or blinks very little, that is a sign of an overly yang condition and a tendency toward mental inflexibility. In terms of constitution, men and women are opposite: for a man, smaller eyes show greater mental clarity, while for a woman, larger eyes show greater mental clarity.

6. The eyebrows show mental tolerance, patience, and endurance. Short eyebrows indicate a short temper, while long eyebrows show a patient, kind, understanding nature. The angle, thickness, and length of individual hairs also show different aspects of that person's mental understanding and sensitivity.

7. The temples show mental development or intellect: a well-developed, prominent temple area indicates a large, well-developed intellectual capacity; small, receding temples show a smaller intellect. By "intellect," I do not mean things like knowledge, college education and mechanical memory; this true intellect is like a detailed, penetrating mental grasp of the universe and various phenomena.

Mental qualities also appear in the horizontal dimensions of the body. For example, if the most indented, narrow part of the torso is tight, this shows a certain type of mental character, and if that is looser or expanded, that also reflects the mind. A person's chest may be wide or narrow, or may come out prominently or recede, while the feet may be flat or arched, narrow or wide, or may go straight or crooked; they may also be flexible or rigid. All these traits are showing something about the person's mental qualities.

Mental discipline appears in the area around the navel, and also corresponds to the mouth. If this area is tight and has good tone, that shows strong self-control; you can see when a person begins to lose his self-control, that area becomes expanded or flabby. Where can we see general mental structure, also corresponding to the jaw? This appears in the shoulders; like the jaw, the shoulders may be wide and prominent or small and receding, indicating a larger or smaller mind. Also like the jaw, there are three general types of shoulders: straight, square shoulders, rounded shoulders, and steeply sloping, almost triangular shoulders, corresponding to the same three mental qualities as those types of jaw. Many people may think that broad, square shoulders are ideal; actually, I would say that if anything is ideal, it would be slightly rounded shoulders, indicating a harmonious, balanced character.

When you see someone from the front, he may have a certain expression on his face that masks his true feelings or true mind; but if you judge by looking at him from behind, the back of the shoulders always reveal the true mind. When you see his smile, you may think he is happy; but from the back he cannot hide—when he turns around to leave the room, you may see that his shoulders give you a sad, lonely feeling. Or, someone may appear flexible and reasonable from the front, but from seeing the back of his neck, head, and shoulders, you can see that he is secretly harboring very stubborn, rigid opinions.

If you see someone from behind and his shoulders appear weak, showing no vitality, even if he appears reasonably healthy from the front, you can be relatively sure that he is developing some type of sickness. By the same token, you can see from behind if a person's shoulders and neck reveal a character that is full of energy, positive mentality, and success.

The feet show a person's mental flexibility, whether wide or narrow; or you might say, mental capacity. The hands also show this: if the hands are flexible and fluid, this shows a character that is good for artistic, aesthetic, invisible, spiritual things. A solid, strong, well-set hand is better for material things, such as business, or practical things like farming and carpentry.

Actually, the hand can also show us a tremendous range of information about a person's state of mind; the hands communicate the entire personality. For example, when you see a conductor conducting a choir, you can tell so many things about his state of mind and his physical health from the sound the choir is making, because all of those things are transmitted to them through the movement of his hands.

Diagnosis of Handwriting

In everyday life, the most practical way to see the movement of a person's hands in detail is through that person's handwriting. As an exercise in this diagnosis, please write down one sentence, and then have several friends each write the same sentence, so you can compare several examples.

You can see so many things from these examples; for instance, you can see which person is more yang, in general, and which is more yin. You can also see the type of character there, whether courageous or timid, inwardly directed or outward, indecisive or confident, artistic or practical, and so on. Also, you can see which organs are the weakest, and what types of food that person likes to eat.

However, to simplify this diagnosis, you can summarize by drawing two lines, one connecting the tops of all the letters and one connecting the bottoms. The first thing you can see is whether these lines are generally orderly or fluctuate way up and down; this corresponds both to the person's general metabolism, and to his general mood, temper, emotions, and sense of order. Now physically speaking, what do these lines show?

These lines show the stream of the hand; they also show the stream of the mind, or stream of consciousness. Physically, they also show the stream of blood through the circulatory system. The upper, yin line shows the path of white blood cells streaming through the body; the yang lower line shows the stream of red blood cells. A strong, even flow of white blood cells shows that that person's antibacterial or biological self-protective mechanism is strong; in other words, he does not easily become sick. An even, regular streaming of red blood cells shows that all the parts of the body are receiving relatively even, strong nourishment and charge from the bloodstream.

Also within the handwriting, all downward lines are more or less showing qualities of the digestive system; all upward lines are showing the condition of the nervous system; connective lines and horizontal lines are showing the character of the circulatory and respiratory functions. Sometimes handwriting is squeezed together, showing that the liver is tight from excessive yang; or you may feel it is loose and open, showing that the stomach is swollen or the large intestine is too loose and watery.

In order to see the principle of detecting various organ troubles in handwriting, we can use a simpler example. Please have your friends draw a simple circle on a piece of paper, and draw one yourself. Since all our organs are related to each other's activities and conditions in a cyclic flow of energy, all of the organs' energies come into play when we draw a simple circle with our hand. If you see someone who can draw a nearly perfect circle, without having to concentrate too hard, just drawing normally, then you can tell that person's organs are all working in harmony.

A circle shows a cycle of movement or energy. When you are beginning to draw downward, moving toward the lower area of the circle, you are using what we call soil energy. This type of energy is correlating with your stomach, spleen, and pancreas. As you reach toward the bottom, that fully gathered, heavy energy corresponds to the lungs and large intestine, or metal energy. Then, as you begin to curve around the bottom and go toward drawing upward, that floating, transitional stage uses water energy, reflecting the condition of the kidneys, bladder, and sex organs. Upward motion is reflecting the liver and gallbladder, or tree energy; and as you reach the highest part of the circle, that fully expanded, active energy shows the condition of the heart, small intestine, triple heater and heart governor, or fire energy.

In other words, when you draw a circle you are creating a perfect picture of your organs' and meridians' conditions according to the diagram of the five transformations. If one part of the circle bulges, then you know that corresponding organ is yin and expanded; if another part of the circle is too tight and not smoothly rounded, that organ is tight and contracted. If some part is shaky or weak, then you can tell that same condition is characteristic of that organ.

Also, you have to see which direction that circle is drawn, so you can know which side was drawn with a descending line and which side was drawn with an ascending line. The particular place where a person begins his drawing also has some certain meaning, which you can figure out. In general, yang people tend to begin at the bottom, while yin people tend to begin at the top.

Even in cases where you do not have an example of actual handwriting, you can find so much information from even simple lines, circles, or figures that someone has drawn, provided you creatively, imaginatively, and accurately apply the principle of yin and yang.

Speaking and Writing

Now, let us consider the difference between writing and speaking. Between these two types of expression, which is more yang? Speaking is using audible vibrations, which are more yang than the short wave visual images your writing produces. Speaking also uses your mouth, the end of your digestive system, while your fingers, which you use for writing, represent an extension of your nervous system. So generally, speaking is a yang form of expression, while writing is yin. Actually, it is difficult to command both of these talents. Usually people who are good speakers do not make such good writers, while those who are eloquent and forceful in their writing tend to be less effective speakers.

For example, George Ohsawa, the founder of modern macrobiotics, wanted to write and speak well, and worked throughout his life to perfect both types of expression. And he was a fine writer—but he could never become a really good speaker. Even at the age of seventy, after decades of experience and tremendous knowledge about yin and yang, when he would get up to talk in front of an audience, his speaking was awkward for the first ten minutes. After that he would become fluent, but it always took great effort.

George Ohsawa had a yin constitution. He was born in October, a yin month; and when you read the poetry he wrote when he was twenty, you can see it is sentimental and yin; delicate and sensitive. Then throughout his life, he tried hard to make himself yang; he plunged into intensive, yang business activities, subjected himself to cold and physical hardship, and took a great amount of salt in his food.

And in many ways, all of this hammering did make him a much more yang person; and he did become proficient at yang disciplines like science, industry, business, and so forth. Yet, inside he never lost that yin, sensitive nature. Once while he was staying at my home, we were talking over dinner with Dr. Neven Henaff, the scientist who was involved in our atomic transmutation research described in the book, *Other Dimensions: Exploring the Unexplained* (Garden City Park, New York: Avery Publishing Group, 1992). Dr. Henaff was about fifty at the time, yet he was still single; so I said, quite naturally, "Dr. Henaff, why are you still single? Don't you miss being with a woman; wouldn't you like to get married?"

He blushed a little bit and muttered something; but late that evening when I was alone with Mr. Ohsawa, he said to me, "Michio, you are so yang! I cannot comprehend how you could say such a thing to him!" For me, that was just normal conversation, but to Mr. Ohsawa that was a very embarrassing episode! So it was difficult for him to speak to someone in person, although he tried to develop that ability; instead, when he wrote about people or directly to people, it was easy for him to point out a person's shortcomings and offer suggestions. But when he would speak, it was difficult for him to say such things.

These examples are only to give you an idea of the unlimited scope of real macrobiotic diagnosis; what I have presented so far, like basic physiognomy, is something like this: before you enter a room, you have to open a door; before you open the door, you must turn the doorknob. Your basic study of physiognomy is something like turning the doorknob—then when you begin to discover these things yourself, that is like opening the door wider and wider. When you are able to actively apply all your growing understanding throughout society, then you are actually entering that room.

When you encounter sick people in the future, you will probably come up against problems that are difficult to figure out. According to your ability in diagnosis, however, you should already know, from the beginning, what kind of mentality the person has, what kind of character he has, what his capacity is to follow your advice, and so forth. In other words, you need to see not only what advice to give, and how to give it, but, from the beginning, you need to take into consideration how well he will be able to practice your recommendations. So, if you sense that he cannot follow your dietary recommendations properly, then you might adjust those recommendations to include more fresh fruit, or in some cases some fish, or you may suggest some kind of gradual schedule he can follow for slowly progressing toward the kind of eating that would be best for him. In other words, macrobiotic diagnosis is not only for symptoms and treatment, but embraces the person's entire life, including his past, present, and future.

Diagnosis of the Pulses

In Chapter 1, we introduced the five stages of energy transformation. Within this cycle, there are two general processes, a yang, contracting process and a yin, expanding process. Within these two general processes, we can differentiate five general stages of change: energy that is solidifying, energy that is heavily materialized and dense, energy that is beginning to dissolve and go toward expansion, energy that is very much evaporating and going up, expanding, and energy that is expanded and active, like free energy.

When we examine the Ki flow of the meridians and their activity, we see that the different energies of each can be characterized according to the five transformations. The liver and gall

Diagnosing the Pulses

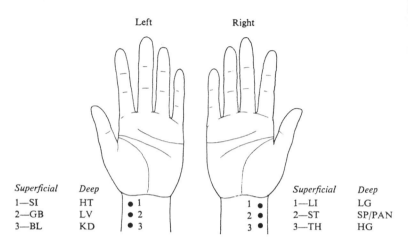

Left			Right		
Superficial	*Deep*			*Superficial*	*Deep*
1—SI	HT	● 1	1 ●	1—LI	LG
2—GB	LV	● 2	2 ●	2—ST	SP/PAN
3—BL	KD	● 3	3 ●	3—TH	HG

The pulses illustrated are for men. In women, the hands are reversed: the pulses shown on the left male wrist are found on the right wrist in females and the pulses shown on the right wrist appear on the left wrist in females.

bladder (LV/GB) correspond to upward, or tree energy, as shown in the diagram. The heart and small intestine (HT/SI) represent actively expanding or fire energy, as do the heart governor and triple heater functions (HG/TH). Downward, or soil energy characterizes the spleen, pancreas, and stomach (SP-PAN/ST), while the lungs and large intestine (LG/LI) correspond to condensed or metal energy. The kidneys and bladder (KD/BL) are represented by floating, or water energy.

The flow of Ki through each of these meridians appears in the pulses on the wrist. Meridians belonging to yin processes appear on the pulses of the left hand, while the yang process meridians appear on the pulses of the right hand. However, as we see in the diagram, the arrangement of the pulses is the not the same for men and women.

The standard arrangement of left and right appears in the old Chinese classics of Oriental medicine; but as people gathered experience, they started to wonder whether or not the pulses are opposite for men and for women. Currently, about 95 percent of Oriental medicine doctors follow the classical way, while a small percent take the pulses on the opposite hands for women and for men. I agree with the opinion that the pulses appear on opposite hands for men and for women. If you hold a pendulum over a man's right and left hands, and then do the same with a woman, you will discover that their energy flow is the opposite. When we take the pulses, we are detecting this opposite flow of energy.

The Relativity of Yin and Yang

In order to see how the pulses appear in the way they do, we need to understand which meridians are yang and which are yin. Let us consider the stomach and spleen as an example. We usually say the stomach is hollow, empty, so that is yin, in terms of structure. The spleen is solid, dense, and compact, so its structure is yang. However, we can also see this in the opposite way, in terms of energy or activity: the stomach is freely, actively moving, so we can say its activity is yang; the spleen does not move much, so we can say it is yin, or less active. Why is the stomach active? Because the meridian that is nourishing it is active—we can call the stomach meridian a yang meridian, and the spleen meridian a yin meridian.

Always remember that yin and yang are relative; there is no absolute yin, and no absolute yang. For example, ice is hard, so we can say structurally it is yang. However, in terms of temperature, it is cold, in other words, yin. If something were yin only, it would expand until it became infinitely large and disappeared. Again, if something were yang only, it would contract until it became infinitely small and disappeared from the phenomenal world. As long as a phenomenon exists, it is inevitably carrying both yin and yang tendencies in some kind of dynamic balance.

Another way to say this is: yin and yang is always a matter of comparison and definition. Whether you are defining yin and yang by comparing structure, by comparing function or activity, or comparing form, or temperature, or chemical reaction, all these different methods of comparison and definition produce different classifications of yin and yang.

If you are seeing yin and yang as an absolute concept, like this is always yin, or that is always yang, then you are making a great mistake. That is not reality, that is only your conceptual rigidity. Actually you should strive to have a very relative, dynamic concept of yin and yang. There are no words to really accurately describe this kind of conception in our modern language, and you cannot learn it in schools or books; to understand this, you really have to change your thinking. It is easy for contradictory interpretations of yin and yang to arise. And often, both explanations can be right at the same time; you only have to differentiate which type of classification you are using for that particular application.

Oriental doctors classify the organs in terms of their activity or function, while in macrobiotics we usually talk in terms of the structure of the organs. So when macrobiotic students study at a school of Chinese medicine, they sometimes get confused: according to Oriental medicine, the stomach is yang, but according to macrobiotics, it is yin—which way is correct? It is important to understand that either way is correct; it all depends upon the application or criteria you are using.

In evaluating cancer, for example, hollow, yin organs tend to have cancer more from excessive yin foods; so the stomach, which is structurally yin, is more susceptible to yin cancer, particularly the most expanded part of the stomach. If this kind of yin cancer arises, then that person needs to eat the standard macrobiotic diet, with a slight emphasis toward yang factors, such as slightly saltier miso soup, slightly more root vegetables, little or no salad, and so on. For that application, our classification in terms of structure works well.

For understanding the pulses of acupuncture, however, that classification by structure may be somewhat confusing; classification in terms of activity works much more efficiently. In this classification, we consider the hollow organs and their meridians to be yang and active, and the compact organs and their meridians to be less active and yin.

Superficial and Deep Pulses

Within these pulses there are two separate sets of pulses; one set is superficial and the other is deep. The energy of the active organs appears at the surface as the superficial, active pulses. These active, yang meridians are: small intestine, gallbladder, bladder, large intestine, stomach, triple heater. So yang energy, yang meridians, yang activity, all appear in the yang, active pulses. For meridians in which the flow of energy is quiet and slow, we find those energies appearing in six deep, quiet pulses. These meridians are: heart, liver, kidney, lung, spleen, heart governor. Yin energy, yin meridians, less activity, all appear in the yin, quiet pulses. Of course, we can also explain this by the other way of classification: the Ki flow of the structurally yin organs, such as the small intestine, gallbladder, and stomach, appears in a yin, superficial position; while organs that are structurally yang, such as the heart, liver, and kidneys, appear in the yang, deep pulses.

Since everyone is different, the pulses do not appear in exactly the same place on everybody; but in about 90 percent of people, the pulses appear in generally the same place. After much practice, you can begin to detect these individual differences. To practice taking the pulses, find the small bone that is sticking out on the thumb side of the wrist. The middle pulse is located next to this bone on the inside of the arm. The other two pulses are located one finger distance above and one finger distance below the middle pulse. Place your hand under the person's wrist, and curl your fingers up around the other side, letting your fingertips rest on these three places. Use your index, middle, and ring fingers, not the flat part of your fingers but the fingertips.

To detect the superficial pulses, just touch each point lightly, one at a time. If you press down deeply, to the extent that you cannot easily press any further, and before the person experiences pain from the pressure, you should be able to detect the deep pulses. The deep pulses are not so brilliant, but more quiet.

Some people have pulses that go regularly, smoothly, and

peacefully; this kind of even, clean pulse shows a good condition in that meridian and organ. In my experience, this kind of pulse is quite rare today, as most people have trouble in their organs because of eating the modern diet. More often, you detect some kind of irregularity or distinctive nature. For example, a person's pulse may feel hard and rigid, or may feel jumpy and excited, or sometimes irregular, something like a zig-zag. Altogether, using the six superficial pulses and six deep pulses, we can detect about 240 symptoms within the body.

However, in order to do that, your own condition must be very good, so your fingers are clean and sensitive. If you are eating cheese and steak, then beneath the skin of your fingers you are collecting hard, thick fatty deposits; or if you are taking sugar, fruit juice or honey every day, the energy in your fingers is too jumpy and irregular, and may overshadow those delicate shades of energy you are trying to detect. In such cases, you can usually still feel several major differences, but not the full range of subtle differences, so you cannot detect so many symptoms.

Recently modern people are eating more oily foods, sugar, meat, and so forth. As a result, many Oriental doctors are no longer able to detect these delicate shades of pulse. So many of them are now beginning to rely instead on modern technological methods of diagnosis, like blood tests, X rays, blood pressure tests, and so forth, or trying to combine these methods with the traditional way.

But originally, Oriental healers kept their condition clear and healthy; they would see first by visual diagnosis to understand generally what problems were there, then confirm these conclusions by taking pulses, occasionally pushing various points here and there for further confirmation, and then immediately begin treatment. This kind of healer did not need diagnostic equipment: his own body and his own judgment were the only diagnostic equipment he needed.

Today, the people who can really learn to take these pulses are those who are making their condition healthy and clear; in other words, people who eat macrobiotically. However, while you are creating the ideal biological condition as a basis for this skill, you also need much practice and experience, taking many, many different people's pulses.

Usually, even if a person is seriously ill, you can still feel the six superficial pulses, since in most cases, those six meridians are still active. But if this sickness is serious, then among the six deep pulses, some may be difficult to detect. For example, suppose a person has liver cancer, which is very progressed, so that his liver is hard. Because it is difficult for the liver to be active in that condition, the liver meridian begins to stagnate. In such a case, you may feel nothing when you try to take the liver pulse. As another example, suppose a person has several small kidney stones; still you can easily detect a kidney pulse, though the character of that pulse may be hard and rigid, or weak. But suppose these stones become larger and larger; eventually this can inhibit kidney function so that you cannot detect any pulse at all.

Traditionally, Oriental healers said that if four deep pulses are undetectable, they could not treat the patient. They believed the patient to be close to death. When a person's sickness reaches this stage, treatment with acupuncture, moxibustion, or shiatsu cannot help them, nor can modern Western medicine or traditional herbal medicine. The only possibility for recovery lies in a special dietary approach, consisting primarily of special rice cream, with macrobiotic condiments. However, in many cases, even that approach may not be successful.

In my experience, among people in modern society who are carrying on apparently normal lives, many already have one or two dead pulses. Four dead pulses is unusual—people in this condition are usually already bedridden at home or in the hospital; but it is not at all uncommon to find one, two, or even sometimes three dead pulses among people today. When I see people, I normally take pulses on only three or four people out of 100. Ordinarily, I rely primarily on visual diagnosis, diagnosis of aura or vibration, expression, and other methods. On occasion, I find it helpful to use this pulse method for confirmation. I hope all students of holistic health will practice this method and master it, as it may be useful in many situations. Eventually, you can graduate to other methods that you can invent yourself.

The Middle Pulses

When I do take pulses, I usually take not only these superficial and deep pulses, but also a pulse that is just in-between. You can detect this pulse by pressing down beneath the superficial pulse, but not so deep that you feel the deep pulse. This middle pulse is showing the character of the body fluids, such as blood and lymph, that nourish each pair of organs. The flow of fluid nourishment influences the condition of each of the organs. We can also use the pulses to detect various mental states and mental problems that the person is experiencing. The superficial pulses show the person's emotions; the middle pulses show intellect; and the deep pulses show basic vitality, or you may say instinct. If the superficial pulses are jumpy; the person's emotional state may be irregular and confused.

Pulse Diagnosis of Emotion

Each of the organs corresponds to a specific emotional state. If the superficial pulse at the point of water nature (bladder) is troubled; then according to the five transformations and their associated emotions, we know that the person is having some trouble with the emotion fear. If the superficial tree nature pulse (gallbladder) is troubled, then anger easily arises. If the superficial fire nature pulse (small intestine) is troubled, then that person easily becomes excitable, uncontrollably overjoyed or hysterical. Trouble in the superficial metal nature (large intestine) pulse shows melancholy, sadness; trouble in the superficial soil nature (stomach) pulse shows indecisiveness, worry, excessive wandering around and too much thinking. Trouble in the triple heater pulse (again this is fire nature) is again excitability, overjoy.

According to the Ko cycle, whenever we emphasize one type of energy, we naturally also suppress the opposite type of energy. For example, fire nature energy is made up of big yin and big yang, although yin is slightly dominant. So the heart and small intestine, which are lying most directly in the path of the body's primary channel, are strongly energized by both heaven's and earth's forces, making them continually active, and thus effecting the transformation of food into blood in the small intestine, and the circulation of blood throughout the entire body in the heart. Therefore, we call these two organs "fire nature energy activated organs."

What kind of energy contradicts fire nature? The kidneys lie not on this primary channel's path, but opposite, along a horizontal line at the middle of the body; one is slightly more yang, one is slightly more yin, and they are quitely managing our balance between liquids and minerals. What kind of energy is this? This is very small yang and very small yin. So naturally, if we are strengthening this water nature energy, activating very small yang and very small yin, then we are suppressing that strong yin and strong yang fire nature—that type of energy cannot arise.

A person who has excessive fire nature energy is usually joyous, outgoing, and easily excitable; he or she generally appears cheerful and happy. Anger does not easily shake his good mood; melancholy, indecisiveness, or worry cannot touch him. But if he should happen to become frightened of something, this can totally suppress his happiness. So he is easily controlled by fear, or water nature energy. This can happen particularly during what season? During winter. And particularly at what time of day? During the late night. So if that type of cheery, smiling person is home alone at night, if he hears a small sound in the pantry, suddenly the smile vanishes from his face! Also, I am sure you have seen in the movies, there are always ladies who have very active hearts, always talking with high, loud voices. Then when a mouse comes, they all go away screaming.

In the same way, every emotion can be easily overridden by another, opposite emotion, as you can see in the diagram; and this can happen particularly easily at those times of day or during those seasons. You can also use this understanding to do emotional healing: suppose you know a person who is always angry—then you can tell him about something sad that happened, and that can override and temporarily cure his anger. Or if some

The Five Transformations and the Organs, Emotions, and Times of Day and Year

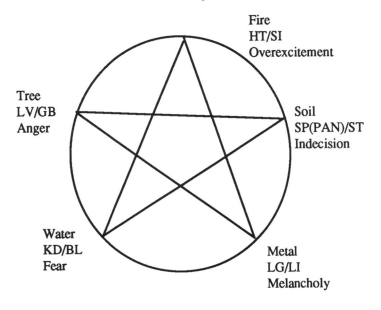

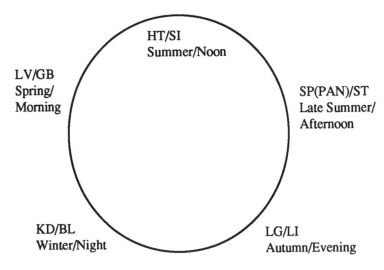

one is sad, then you can give him big joy; and so forth. Now, by taking these six superficial pulses alone, you can already tell so much about a person's emotional condition and what kind of emotional tendencies he or she has, together with the time of day or year these tendencies are strongest. When you practice taking pulses, make your conclusions about that person's emotional state and tendencies, and write these conclusions down in your notes.

Pulse Diagnosis of Intellect and View of Life

Now, let us look at how to interpret the person's intellectual tendencies by using the middle pulses. Looking at each pulse in order, you can interpret these tendencies:

Heart/small intestine—suspense, sense of adventure
Liver/gallbladder—idealism
Kidney/bladder—caution, protectiveness, or cowardice
Lung/large intestine—sensitivity, poetic nature
Spleen/stomach—suspicion
Heart governor/triple heater—exaggeration

If you check these middle pulses and you find one certain pulse is irregular or jumpy, then you know that person tends to be too idealistic, too sensitive, or too suspicious, or it may be he is unable to be sensitive, or unable to be idealistic, or unable to exercise normal caution.

Next, let us see how to interpret the deep pulses; these are showing a person's basic vitality, or you may say, that person's basic view of life, or basic life direction. Here are these six tendencies:

Heart—positive lifestyle and outlook, with creative progressive ideas
Liver—self-control, or patience

Kidney—resistance, endurance, tolerance

Lung—broad understanding, comprehension

Spleen—clarity, clear understanding, observation and judgment

Heart governor—sociability, range and pace of social activity

Suppose you find some person who has no deep pulse for the liver, the liver pulse is "dead." Then you know that person has no patience at all. Or suppose some person's sixth deep pulse is irregular: then you know that person's social life is uneven; their basic way of life does not presently have a strong or normal social component. When you practice taking pulses, do so with a view toward these various tendencies. Compare your observations with the above. Then talk over these conclusions with the person, and verify whether you were right or wrong. Perhaps you were right and he was not even aware of those tendencies.

To really have a good beginning grasp of these pulses, you should check several different people, in this same thorough way, comparing all your conclusions and also discussing them with each person. Then you will begin to really see how accurately and beautifully these simple ways of diagnosis can show us so many things about a person's life. In the following table, we have summarized all three of these types of tendencies: superficial pulses and emotions, middle pulses and intellectual tendencies, deep pulses and basic mentality, or view of life.

Interpretation of the Eighteen Pulses

Organ/ Meridian	Superficial Pulse	Middle Pulse	Deep Pulse
	(emotion)	(intellect)	(view of life)

Man's Left / Woman's Right

Fire (HT/SI)	Overjoy Excitability	Suspense Adventure	Positive Creative
Tree (LV/GB)	Anger	Idealism	Self-control Patience
Water (KD/BL)	Timidity Fear	Caution Protectiveness	Endurance Tolerance

Man's Right / Woman's Left

Metal (LG/LI)	Grief Melancholy	Sensitivity Poetic	Broad understanding, comprehension
Soil	Worry Indecision	Suspicion	Clarity of observation and judgment
Fire (HG/TH)	Overjoy Excitability	Exaggeration	Sociability

Conclusion

There is so much we can learn and figure out from the ancient, holistic techniques of Oriental philosophy and medicine. If you are content with just learning what you can find out from *The Yellow Emperor's Classic of Internal Medicine* and acupuncture, you should know that this information is only just scratching the surface of what you can see about the human condition: for that human condition, while appearing small and insignificant, actually has infinite depth. Also, in my own books, lectures, and seminars, I have presented only a small fraction of what I have learned—and I am certain that what I have learned is only the tip of an infinite iceberg. So please do not be content with knowing only a tiny fraction; I hope through your continuing study and practice, your understanding of diagnosis will extend far beyond this basic level.

6
Macrobiotic Diet

What is food? That question is very important for our understanding of life and health, and for our practice of healing. Before we answer this question, however, let us first consider another question: which has prior existence, food or humanity? Do we eat food, or is food becoming us? Without food, we would not be here. Our hair, brain cells, any part of our body, what were they originally? They were food. Food exists prior to or before human life, and food becomes or changes into human life.

The biological world exists immediately prior to us. We are part of the biological world, which we divide into the animal and vegetable kingdoms. And before that is the world of nature—air, water, land, and sea. Then before that is the world of small particles and waves. That world creates and maintains the elements of nature, and the elements eventually return to that world. Light is like that: a small particle and a wave. Electrons, protons, and other subatomic particles are in this world. What creates the particles of the preatomic world? The world of vibration. Vibrations come in various forms: some with long waves, others short; some with positive charges, other with negative. All vibrations are created by two primary energies, yin and yang, or expansion and contraction, that arise in the ocean of the infinite universe.

Does infinity exist in pure form somewhere? No. Infinity exists in relative form. You have relative existence. The sun, moon, stars, and planets all have relative existence. The invisible, spiritual world also has a relative, not an absolute, existence. Infinity does not appear as absolute; the absolute does not appear as absolute, but in a countless number of changing, relative forms. So relative law, the unifying principle, yin and yang, is the law of absoluteness. If you know the laws and mechanisms of yin and yang, you know the justice of the kingdom of heaven, or the order of infinity itself.

The world of yin and yang creates vibration, which creates the preatomic world, which in turn creates air, water, vegetables, animals, and man. Then what is food? What are animals and vegetables, the seas, land, and atmosphere? They are all food. The preatomic world and world of vibration are also food. Everything, the whole universe, is food; there is nothing but food, and in various ways we are taking in the entire universe. We are not eating in the sense that we are the center and go out and select something to eat. We are here and are eating because these things have always been coming toward us. In other words, eating is the inevitable course of the universe. Eating is not the result of our small will or desire, but the course of the entire universe. The entire universe, through a process of change, becomes food for man and changes into man.

So do not think this way: "I ate this. I'd like to eat that; I am choosing; I am eating." Everything in the universe is moving toward you, and your process of choosing is nothing but the relationship between food and food. Suppose you eat salmon. What do you want to eat after that? Perhaps ice cream. At that time, is it you that wants the ice cream? No, food is wanting other food. You are the phantom of food—yesterday's food, the food of a month ago, the food of four months ago. The food of the past several months, or in some cases, several years, is wanting other food to make balance.

When you think, "I am here," " I have certain abilities," "I'd like to do this or that, be famous, marry so-and-so," that "I" does not exist at all in this universe. It is a conceptual illusion that we call "ego." Buddha, Jesus, and other great healers and spiritual teachers wanted to demolish that ego, that way of thinking. When you demolish that thinking, you awake to the real world.

But nearly everyone is dreaming and seeing illusions, and these illusions are the primary cause of our sickness and unhappiness.

You do not choose the food that goes into your body. The food assembled over several months is seeking other food. When you think you want salmon, in actuality, past food is wanting salmon. Then salmon wants ice cream, and then ice cream wants water. So our body, our existence, our life is nothing but attraction and repulsion between foods: one type of food attracting another type; one volume of food attracting another volume. It is this process of food adjustment that we call eating. The art of adjusting is what we call cooking. When you know the order of eating, including the proper way of cooking, you know practically this entire universe.

Food Ratios

There are various kinds of food, including foods of animal and vegetable origin, together with air, water, vibration, and minerals. The key to understanding the order of food is to understand the ratios that govern our intake of these different parts of our environment, and the key to discovering these ratios is the logarithmic spiral. Logarithmic spirals can be of various ratios. Our universe has the form of a gigantic logarithmic spiral with a ratio of one to seven. In drawing it, we would place the first intersection on the right at one, the next would come at seven points from the center on the left; the next at forty-nine units from the center on the right, and so on. If we were drawing this on a blackboard, that point would reach across the room. Logarithmic ratios occur throughout nature.

Consider the creation of the vegetable kingdom. The most recent vegetable species to appear were the cereal grains. Of these, there are five major types: rice, wheat, rye, millet, and barley. Corn and buckwheat are not true cereals, although they are closely related to the cereal grains and can be used as substitutes. Each of these five major branches has hundreds of varieties. Fruits are one step removed from cereal grains. Here there are thirty-five major branches, or seven times five, each with many varieties. Leafy vegetables come next, and in this world, there are seven times thirty-five, or 245 major branches. The plant kingdom developed in the form of a logarithmic spiral, with cereal grains as the center, the end result.

In general, we take in nourishment in a logarithmic ratio of one to seven. This balance enables us to maintain harmony with the environment, and is reflected in the proportion of major nutrients we consume. In general, we need to consume seven times more protein than minerals. When people eat boiled eggs, for example, which are comprised mostly of protein and fat, they usually put salt on them; otherwise they have little taste. Salt supplies the necessary minerals, thus maintaining the one to seven ratio between minerals and protein. It is difficult to eat salt or protein by themselves. If you wish to eat salt, you need to balance it with seven times more protein.

Then, in order to balance our environment, we need to take in seven times more carbohydrate than protein. If you eat steak or hamburger, you naturally want to follow it with dessert or sweets. Meat, poultry, and other high-protein foods attract seven times more fruit or other source of sugar; if you eat these foods and do not balance them with carbohydrates, you lose harmony with the environment. Then further, we are attracted to seven times more water than carbohydrate. In daily food, the ratio between solid and liquid averages out to one to seven. The water we take in is not necessarily consumed as beverage, since water already exists in solid foods. When you drink a sweet liquid such as apple cider, you may become thirsty afterward. Apple cider is made up of water and plenty of sugar, but not in a ratio of seven to one; the amount of sugar is higher. If the ratio between sugar and water were one to seven, it would be satisfactory. It is the need to balance this additional sugar that makes you thirsty. The same is true of alcohol. People often become thirsty and crave water after drinking alcoholic beverages.

The next form of food, air, is taken in a much larger volume than water. The ratio between our intake of air and our intake of water is generally seven to one. We normally eat solid foods—

minerals, proteins, carbohydrates, and fats—several times per day. We take water more frequently, in a volume that is about seven times greater than the amount of solid food. Air is taken constantly. The humidity in the air is constantly changing; sometimes it is 70 percent, sometimes 30 percent. When it reaches 100 percent, it begins to rain. When the humidity becomes very high, we do not need to drink much, because we absorb water from the air through our lungs. When it is very dry, we need to drink more.

Vibrations or waves exist in abundance beyond the earth's atmosphere. The ratio between our intake of air and our intake of vibration is also one to seven. We are constantly absorbing vibrations from the environment, both near and far. Yin and yang, or the primary forces of expansion and contraction, are the source of all vibration. However, yin and yang are tendencies, not phenomena. The thing that we take in in a volume that is seven times greater than vibration is the force of infinity itself. All vibrations take the form of waves, some with short and others with longer wavelengths. Infinite force does not take the form of waves; it moves in a straight line at infinite speed. Motion at infinite speed erases time and space, so in the absolute world, space and time do not exist. We can think of this aspect of food as having the form of infinitely expanding force.

The Energy of Food

As we saw in Chapter 3, daily foods, like everything else in nature, can be understood in terms of yin and yang. Eggs, meat, cheese, chicken, fish, seafood, and other animal products produce heat and constriction. They represent the concentration of a great deal of plant food, are rich in hemoglobin, and contain hard, saturated fat. On the other hand, vegetable foods have a cooling and relaxing effect. They are rich in chlorophyll and the oil they contain is usually lighter, less dense, and unsaturated. On the whole, animal foods have more yang or contractive energy while vegetable foods, including grains, beans, seeds, and fruits, are more yin or expansive. A wide range of variation exists within these two categories of foods. Some animal foods are more contractive than others. Within the realm of animal life, including fish, shellfish, birds, reptiles, and mammals, inactive or slow-moving species are usually more yin than fast-moving, active species. A slow-moving carp, therefore, would be more yin than a fast-moving bluefish or tuna, while an octopus, which moves slowly through the water, is more yin than a rapidly darting shrimp. Cold-blooded species such as fish and shellfish, which are less biologically developed, are more yin than more highly evolved warm-blooded species. Also, species that live in cold climates are generally yang in comparison to those in warm regions, as are species that live on dry land in comparison to aquatic species.

Climate plays an important role in determining the nature of energy in plant foods. A colder, more yin climate produces plants with smaller, more compact structures. A warmer, more yang climate makes vegetation develop a more expanded form. Northern plants are thus more yang, while tropical species, including fruits such as pineapples, bananas, and grapefruit, are juicier, more acidic, and yin. Thus avocados, which grow in warm regions, are more yin than squash or cabbage grown in the north. Vegetables that were grown initially in the tropics and transplanted in the north, such as tomatoes, potatoes, and eggplant, are also very yin.

The seasonal cycle also plays an important role in determining the type of energy in a food. Vegetables that grow in spring or summer, such as summer squash, lettuce, and Chinese cabbage, are more yin than fall or winter varieties such as fall squash, kale, and watercress. Foods that are more yin have a stronger charge of earth's rising energy; foods that are more yang are more strongly charged by heaven's contracting force. However, all foods have both yin and yang energies; this classification is based on which of the two forces is predominant.

Animal Foods

Eggs are the compact essence of new life, and are generally the most yang among animal foods. Smaller eggs, such as those laid by wild birds, are more yang than larger varieties. Eggs that are fertilized and produced by organically-fed chickens are more yang than those produced by chickens kept in artificial environments and fed hormones and antibiotics. Meat is a more yang food; drier and less fatty varieties more so than those which are moist and high in fat. Poultry and fish are less yang than meat, with low-fat, white-meat fish generally the least yang among them. Dry, salty cheeses are yang, while milk and cottage cheese, which are watery and have a sweeter taste, are more yin. Modern commercial yogurts, especially those processed with fruit and sugar, are very yin or expansive, as is ice cream.

Whole Cereal Grains and Beans

Whole grains represent the fusion of fruit and seed in one compact unit and occupy the center of the food spectrum. Whole grains come closest to reflecting the seven to one ratio between heaven's and earth's forces that exists on planet earth, and this is reflected in their ratio of minerals to proteins to carbohydrates. The complex carbohydrates in grains are made up of many small molecules of glucose that are held together by strong contracting energy. In contrast, simple sugars are more yin and are composed of many loose molecules of glucose. They lack the cohesiveness of complex carbohydrates and produce more extreme yin effects in the body.

Complex carbohydrates are also found in beans, vegetables, and sea vegetables. They require thorough chewing to be digested properly. Because they are more yang, they are slowly broken down and not absorbed until they reach the small intestine. They provide a steady source of energy in contrast to simple sugars, which bypass the normal digestive process and are rapidly absorbed into the bloodstream. Although whole grains are centrally balanced in terms of yin and yang energies, certain varieties are more strongly expansive, and others more contractive. Buckwheat grows in cold, northern climates and is more yang, while corn, which grows in warm, sunny climates, is more yin. Brown rice and whole wheat are generally in the middle, with wheat being somewhat more yin than rice. Short grain rice is generally the most balanced of the main varieties of rice. Medium and long grain rice grow in warmer climates and are more yin than short grain rice.

Beans are usually larger and more expanded than grains and are higher in fat and protein. They have more yin energy than grains. Azuki and other small, low-fat varieties of beans are more yang than lima, pinto, and other beans that are larger and higher in fat.

Vegetables

On the whole, vegetables are more yin than grains and beans, but again, a wide range of variation is found among them. Burdock root, carrots, turnips and other root vegetables are more yang; cabbage, squash, onions, and other vegetables with round shapes are in-between; and expanded leafy vegetables, such as mustard greens and Chinese cabbage, are more yin.

Yin and yang variations exists within each of these categories. If you compare the size, shape, and structure of mustard greens to that of carrot, daikon, or turnip tops, you will notice that the green tops of these root vegetables have smaller leaf structures. Each leaf is small and more finely differentiated than the broader leaves of the mustard plant. The green tops of root vegetables have more yang or contracting energy than greens with broader shapes. Because of their high mineral content, many varieties of sea vegetables are more yang or contractive than land vegetables, especially those that grow deeper in the ocean or in cold regions.

Seeds, Nuts, and Fruits

Seeds and nuts, which are higher in fat and oil than grains or beans, are generally more yin or expansive. Between the two, nuts—which are oilier—are more yin than most varieties of seeds. Low-fat seeds such as pumpkin are more yang, while sunflower seeds are higher in oil and are more yin. Cashews, Brazil nuts, and other tropical nuts are more oily, yin, and expansive than walnuts, chestnuts, and other temperate varieties.

On the whole, fruits are more expansive than the types of vegetables we have discussed above. For the most part, they are juicier, grow mostly in warmer seasons, decompose rapidly, contain fructose, a form of simple sugar, and are acidic. Fruits that grow in northern latitudes are more yang than those grown in warmer or tropical zones. Strawberries, berries, and other small fruits are generally more yang than melons or larger fruits, while varieties that grow in trees are more yin than those growing on or near the ground.

Sweeteners, Tropical Foods, and Drugs and Medications

Concentrated sweeteners such as refined sugar, honey, and maple syrup are very yin or expansive. Refined sugar is the most extreme of these substances. Artificial sweeteners are also extremely yin. Concentrated sweeteners derived from the complex carbohydrates in whole grains—such as brown rice syrup and barley malt—are less yin than sweeteners that come from the simple sugars in sugar cane or maple sap. Like cane sugar, foods such as coffee, spices, and chocolate come from tropical zones. They are all strongly yin. Alcohol is also an extremely yin substance, as are most drugs and medications, including antibiotics, aspirin, cortisone, and illicit drugs such as marijuana and cocaine. The artificial fertilizers and insecticides used by modern agriculture are also strongly yin, as are the growth hormones used in the livestock industry and many of the additives used in modern food processing.

Cooking and Food Processing

Cooking and food processing change the energy of foods and beverages. Fire, pressure, salt, and time (aging) cause foods to become more yang or contracted. On the other hand, using little or no pressure, adding water or oil, or using fresh foods makes our diet become more yin. Cooking and food processing employ these complementary influences in varying degrees, in order to rebalance the energy of food, and if they are managed properly, to create harmony with the environment and with our needs and preferences.

Classifying Foods

Another way to understand the energy of food is to classify foods into three categories: (1) foods with strong yang energy, (2) foods with strong yin energy, and (3) foods with a moderate combination of both energies. Strong yang and strong yin foods are best avoided for optimal health in a temperate climate, while foods with an even balance of both energies are recommended for regular consumption. The foods in the strong yang column are primarily animal foods and are naturally eaten in higher proportions in colder regions of the world. The foods in the strong yin column are mostly vegetable foods and are mostly native to the tropics. The centrally balanced foods in the middle column are common to the temperate zones.

The modern diet is based mostly on foods from the strong yang category and the strong yin category. Historically, most of these foods originated in either colder northern climates or in hotter southern climates, even though they are now produced in temperate zones owing to the development of modern technology. In their original habitats, some of these foods are part of a balanced natural diet, for example, curry and spices in India, coconuts in the Pacific Islands, and meat and dairy food in Siberia and Alaska. However, when consumed on a regular basis in a

The Three Categories of Food

Strong Yang Foods
Refined Salt
Eggs
Meat
Poultry
Seafood
Fish

More Balanced Foods
Whole Cereal Grains
Beans and Bean Products
Root, Round, and Leafy Green Vegetables
Sea Vegetables
Unrefined Sea Salt, Vegetable Oil, and Other Seasonings
Spring and Well Water
Nonaromatic, Nonstimulant Teas and Beverages
Seeds and Nuts
Temperate-Climate Fruit
Rice Syrup, Barley Malt, and Other Grain-Based Natural
    Sweeteners

Strong Yin Foods
White Rice, White Flour
Frozen and Canned Foods
Tropical Fruits and Vegetables
Milk, Cream, Yogurt, and Ice Cream
Refined Oils
Spices (pepper, curry, nutmeg, etc.)
Aromatic and Stimulant Beverages (coffee, black tea, etc.)
Honey, Sugar, and Refined Sweeteners
Alcohol
Foods Containing Chemicals, Preservatives, Dyes, Pesticides
Drugs (marijuana, cocaine, etc. with some exceptions)
Medications (tranquilizers, antibiotics, etc. with some
    exceptions

four-season climate, strong yin and strong yang foods are unnatural and create sickness and imbalance.

As we will see below, it is important when eating for optimal health to base your diet on foods from your own climate or one that is similar to yours. Therefore, if you live in the temperate zones, eating avocados, pineapples, mangoes, and other tropical fruits results in imbalance, as does including vegetables such as tomatoes, potatoes, eggplant, and other members of the nightshade family that originated in the equatorial zones before being imported to Europe and North America.

Yin and yang attract one another like man and woman or the oppositely charged poles of a magnet. When we eat plenty of foods with extreme yang energy we are inevitably attracted to yin extremes, and vice versa. This extreme pattern prevails today, and is a major factor in the widespread incidence of degenerative conditions. When the diet is based on extremes, the body is forced to cope with unnecessary excessive factors, including saturated fat, cholesterol, simple sugar, and chemical additives. Moreover, foods high in fat, cholesterol, and refined sugar tend to displace nutritious, centrally balanced grains, beans, and fresh local vegetables. Overall balance is much harder to maintain, and we lose harmony with our environment and our health and well-being.

Macrobiotic Principles

Macrobiotics is the natural way of life for humanity. It is predicated on the unchanging laws of nature. In the macrobiotic definition, food includes not only the substances we consume through dietary practice, but the whole scope of environmental factors we consume in various ways. This definition includes minerals, as a part of the inorganic world; liquid, as part of the water environment covering the earth; air, as a part of the atmosphere surrounding the earth; and vibrations, waves, rays, and various forms of radiation, as a part of our universe.

Human well-being cannot be achieved if we do not maintain

the proper balance between these environmental factors, simply because human life is a part of the planetary environment which is in turn a part of the universe. Our daily requirement for these components fluctuates with personal needs, climatic conditions, social activities, age and sex differences. However, according to the current evolutionary stage of the planet, the ideal ratio by weight between these components fluctuates between one to five and one to ten, with the average proportion being one to seven. As we saw above, these ratios can be stated as follows:

Mineral to protein: standard one to seven by weight;
Protein to carbohydrate: standard one to seven by weight;
Carbohydrate to water: standard one to seven by weight;
Water to air: standard one to seven by weight;
Air to vibration: standard one to seven by weight.

During the different stages of planetary evolution, there have been corresponding stages of biological evolution. These ratios have been changing, due to the change of centrifugal forces going out from the earth as it rotates and the centripetal forces coming in toward the center of the earth from outer space, including cosmic rays, radiation, waves, and other forms of vibration. Human beings are the latest development in the biological world. They are a product of recent planetary conditions, including a ratio between centrifugal and centripetal forces (the force from the earth and the force from heaven) that averages one to seven. Thus the one to seven ratio can be found in the human form, for example, in the average size of the head and the width of the waist to the height of the body as a whole. We also see this ratio reflected in the traditional dietary practices of cultures around the world.

The primary food that has contributed to the appearance and development of the human species has been the cereal grains, which, when unrefined, generally maintain the one to seven ratio between minerals and protein, and protein and carbohydrate. In order to achieve the proper one to seven balance between carbohydrates and water, water is added to the grains during the process of cooking. Cooking began in an unknown prehistoric age, and helped facilitate the smooth transformation of plant foods into human blood and cells, and the smooth release of the energy stored in grains and vegetables. The art of cooking contributed to the advancement of human species toward homo sapiens.

For this reason, whole cereal grains, such as brown rice, whole wheat, barley, rye, and millet should be our main daily food, with corn and buckwheat serving as substitutes depending upon climatic and geographical conditions. Though this substitution may be extended to include other foods such as beans, foods other than cereal grains should not become the central foods in the human diet.

Other kinds of food, including land and sea vegetables and various types of animal food, are appropriate as supplements to our primary food, which should be whole cereal grains. If these supplemental foods are used as primary foods in the daily diet, our physical and mental condition easily becomes unbalanced and disharmonious in relation to our environment on earth. At the present time, various types of nutritional advice, including many conflicting opinions, are creating a great deal of confusion. This is due to the fact that the role of cereal grains in the biological accomplishment of human beings has been almost completely forgotten.

It is important to maintain order in the selection of supplementary foods of both vegetable and animal sources, keeping in mind not only the analytical view of nutrient balance, but also a larger view based on the following considerations.

Biological Evolution

All forms of life on earth have evolved because of environmental change, in combination with their dietary habits. The reason why some species become prosperous, while others diminish is largely due to their dietary habits, with those of the latter being rigid and unable to adapt to changing environmental conditions. Each species, from invertebrates, amphibians, reptiles and birds, mammals, apes, up to and including man has maintained its main food, and the supplementary food of each species has consisted of the primary food of the species that came before it. Human beings can eat anything that existed prior to their appearance on earth, but when choosing supplementary foods from the plant kingdom, it is preferable to eat a larger volume of more recent species and a smaller volume of more remote, ancient ones. This principle can be applied practically as follows:

1. Soup should be a replica of the ancient ocean, and may consist of water, sea salt, enzymes, bacteria, sea vegetables, and/or occasional fish, land vegetables, beans, or grains.
2. Vegetable dishes should consist of a larger volume of modern species and a smaller volume of ancient species.
3. Fruits, nuts, and seeds may be used as supplements in small volume, due to their biological period which, in relation to other plant species, was comparatively short.

From the time of conception, and through the embryonic period into infancy, we depend entirely upon animal food, initially in the form of the nutrients supplied by the mother's bloodstream and then in the form of mother's milk. But after the appearance of the first tooth, together with the upright position of the body, we should begin to eat more vegetable food in order to accomplish further evolution.

Again, due to biological order, the balance between vegetable and animal food should average seven to one by weight. This proportion appears in the formation of human teeth:

28 incisors, premolars, and molars—for grains, beans and vegetables
4 canine teeth — for animal food, in a ratio of seven to one

Climatic and Seasonal Order

In order to balance their climate, people who live in cold polar regions may consume more animal food, while those who live under hot, semitropical climates should depend almost totally upon vegetable foods. People who live in a four-season climate can eat generally in accord with the order of biological evolution, with cereal grains as main foods, and soups and vegetables of land and sea as secondary foods. Fruits, nuts, and seeds can serve as their third source, and animal food which is biologically far removed from the human species, such as fish and other types of seafood, can serve as the fourth supplement.

To adapt to the changes in temperature, humidity, and other atmospheric conditions that come about due to the changing of the seasons, we need to change our selection and manner of cooking daily foods, including cereal grains and supplementary foods:

— In colder seasons, food needs to be cooked more thoroughly and the amount of salt increased slightly.

— In hotter seasons, food can be cooked less, with less salty seasoning added.

— In higher humidity, food can be cooked with less water.

— In lower humidity, food can be cooked with more water.

The various arts and techniques used in cooking need to be applied in a flexible manner to harmonize with the changing of the seasons. The selection of supplementary foods also helps us to adapt to seasonal change, especially when we rely upon foods that are naturally available in each season and that grow in the same or a similar climate.

Geographical Order

Foods are part of the natural environment, and should come primarily from our immediate geographical area. People who live in the mountains should rely mostly upon foods grown in the mountains, and people who live on the plains should depend primarily upon products of the plains. Together with this natural law, certain foods need to be selected from the immediate environment, and certain others can be selected from more distant places, generally as follows:

Air—immediate place
Water—immediate surrounding environment
Fruits—same climatic and geographical area
Vegetables—more extended geographical and climatic area, but similar to the immediate place
Grains and beans—further extended areas, which share the same geographical and similar climatic conditions
Sea vegetables—even further extended area along the same climatic belt
Sea salt—entire hemisphere, either northern or southern, depending upon where people live

However, the above should not be extended to include the opposite hemisphere from which one lives. So, if you live in a four-season climate in the northern hemisphere, you should not import food from the southern hemisphere, and vice versa. This is due to the tremendous difference in atmospheric, oceanic, and electromagnetic conditions between the two hemispheres. These different influences are, in many ways, very subtle and according to present technological review, are largely undetectable.

Personal Modification

Along with the general laws of food described above, personal modifications need to be made, according to such factors as age, sex, tradition, and activity, in addition to social, cultural, and family background. These modifications may appear in the kinds of foods used, as well as in the ways of cooking and combining ingredients to produce a wide variety of attractive and appealing dishes. However, dietary modifications are best made within the general guidelines presented above. If dietary modifications take place outside of these principles, or if these natural laws are ignored, physical and mental disorders arise, either in the form of acute conditions or chronic degenerative conditions.

Proper dietary practice is the main source of health and happiness for both individuals and the community, including the family, nation, and the world. On the other hand, improper dietary practice is a major source of all disorder, including physical disease, mental disturbances, and social conflicts. Holistic medicine, therefore, should depend largely upon the order of eating and consider diet as the major cause of all sorts of disorders, and should discover that the solution to personal and social conditions can be found in the improvement of dietary practice. Not only cardiovascular disorders, cancer, diabetes, skin disease, and many other physical ailments, but also depression, melancholy, schizophrenia, paranoia, along with the physical-psychological causes of violence, crime, and other human difficulties can be solved through the correction of dietary practice.

According to the principles described above, standard dietary practice in a temperate, four-season climate would generally be as follows:

50 to 60 percent whole cereal grains
5 to 10 percent sea vegetable and vegetable soup
20 to 30 percent vegetables, mostly cooked, but sometimes fresh due to necessity
5 to 10 percent beans and sea vegetables

Plus the occasional use of fish and seafood, and fresh, dried, or cooked fruits, nuts, and seeds

Condiments and seasonings are best made from natural sea salt or other natural foods such as fermented soybean products like miso and tamari soy sauce. As much as possible, animal or saturated fats are best avoided, and even unsaturated vegetable oils are best used moderately in seasoning and cooking.

The macrobiotic diet is based on an understanding of the relationship between humanity and the natural environment. Macrobiotic principles can be found in the dietary practice of many traditional religions and cultures. The value of traditional dietary practices should be recognized in this critical age of degeneration. Naturally balanced diet is the primary method for beginning the reconstruction of humanity toward the realization of a healthy and peaceful world. Below are more detailed guidelines for selecting the best foods in a temperate, or four-season climate.

General Guidelines

Standard Macrobiotic Diet

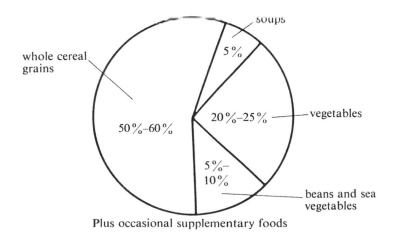

Plus occasional supplementary foods

Whole Cereal Grains

Whole cereal grains are the staff of life and an essential part of a balanced diet for health and healing. They constitute up to 50 to 60 percent of the standard macrobiotic diet. Below is a list of the whole grains and grain products that are frequently included:

Regular Use
Barley
Buckwheat
Corn
Medium grain brown rice
  (in warmer areas or seasons)
Millet
Pearl barley (hato mugi)
Rye
Short grain brown rice
Whole oats
Whole wheat berries
Other traditionally used
  whole grains

Occasional Use
Corn grits
Cornmeal
Couscous
Cracked wheat (bulgur)
Long grain brown rice
Mochi (a cake made from
  pounded sweet brown
  rice)
Rolled oats
Rye, wheat, rice, and other
  whole grain flakes
Steel cut oats

Sweet brown rice
Other traditionally
  used whole grain
  products

Occasional Use
Flour Products
Fu
Seitan
Soba (buckwheat)
  noodles
Somen (thin wheat)
  noodles
Udon (wheat) noodles
Unyeasted whole rye
  bread
Unyeasted whole
  wheat bread
Whole wheat noodles
Other whole grain
  products that were
  used traditionally

Cooked whole grains are preferable to flour products or to cracked or rolled grains because of their easier digestibility. In general, it is better to keep the intake of flour products—or cracked or rolled grains—to less than 15 to 20 percent of your daily consumption of whole grains.

For the improvement of health, it is best to temporarily limit the intake of baked flour products such as cookies, muffins, crackers, chapatis, and so on, even when they are made from whole grain flours. However, natural unyeasted whole grain sourdough bread can be eaten when desired, usually several times per week; whole wheat noodles (udon) can also be included several times per week, preferably in soup or broth.

Persons who have had surgery within the past two years are advised to temporarily avoid buckwheat noodles (soba) and whole buckwheat (kasha), due to the strongly contractive nature of buckwheat and its products. Oatmeal made from rolled or cut oats is also best eaten only on occasion, as are other rolled, milled, or partially refined grains or grain products.

Short grain brown rice is recommended as the primary grain for daily consumption, and pressure cooking is the preferred method for preparing brown rice in a temperate climate. For variety, brown rice can be cooked with grains such as millet, barley, pearl barley (hato mugi), and wheat berries, or with azuki or other beans

Theses ingredients can be cooked in the same dish, using, for example, 80 to 85 percent brown rice and 15 to 20 percent of these other ingredients.

Porridge made from leftover brown rice and other whole grains can be eaten as a hot breakfast cereal. Simply add water to leftover grains and reheat. Corn on the cob, fresh and in season, can also be eaten several times per week, without butter.

Soups

Soups comprise about 5 percent of the standard macrobiotic diet. For most people, that averages out to about one or two cups or small bowls per day. A wide variety of ingredients, including vegetables, grains, beans, sea vegetables, noodles, tofu, tempeh, and, occasionally, white-meat fish can be used in soups. Soups are delicious when moderately seasoned with either miso, tamari soy sauce, sea salt, umeboshi plum or paste, or occasional ginger.

Soups can be made thick and rich, or as simple clear broths. Vegetable, grain, or bean stews can also be enjoyed, while a variety of garnishes, such as scallions, parsley, and nori sea vegetable may be used to enhance the appearance and flavor of soups.

Light miso soup, with vegetables and wakame or kombu, is recommended daily—on the average, one small bowl or cup per day. Mugi (barley) miso is the best for regular consumption, followed by soybean (Hatcho) miso. Miso is processed with natural sea salt, so use it in moderation. Miso soup should have a mild flavor and not be too salty. Change the recipe often. A second cup or bowl of soup may also be enjoyed, preferably mildly seasoned with tamari soy sauce or sea salt. Other healthful varieties of soup include:

Bean and vegetable soups
Puréed squash and other vegetable soups
Grain and vegetable soups

Vegetables

Roughly one-quarter to one-third (25 to 30 percent) of daily intake can include vegetables. Nature provides an incredible variety of fresh local vegetables to choose from. Recommended varieties include:

Regular Use
Acorn squash
Bok choy
Broccoli
Brussels sprouts
Burdock
Butternut squash
Cabbage
Carrots
Carrot tops
Cauliflower
Chinese cabbage
Collard greens
Daikon
Daikon greens
Dandelion greens
Dandelion roots
Hokkaido pumpkin
Hubbard squash
Jinenjo
Kale
Leeks
Lotus root
Mustard greens
Onions
Parsley
Parsnip
Pumpkin
Radish
Red cabbage
Rutabaga
Scallions
Turnip
Turnip greens
Watercress

Occasional Use
Celery
Chives
Coltsfoot
Cucumber
Endive
Escarole
Green beans
Green peas
Iceberg lettuce
Jerusalem artichoke
Kohlrabi
Lamb's-quarters
Mushrooms
Pattypan squash
Romaine lettuce
Salsify
Shiitake mushrooms
Snap beans
Snow peas
Sprouts
Summer squash
Wax beans

Avoid (for optimal health)
Artichoke
Bamboo shoots
Beets
Curly dock
Eggplant
Fennel
Ferns
Ginseng
Green/red pepper
New Zealand spinach

Avoid (continued)

Okra	Sweet potato
Plantain	Swiss chard
Potato	Taro (albi) potato
Purslane	Tomato
Shepherd's purse	Yams
Sorrel	Zucchini
Spinach	

Vegetables can be served in soups, or with grains, beans, or sea vegetables. They can also be used in making rice rolls (homemade sushi), served with noodles or pasta, cooked with fish, or served alone. The most common methods for cooking vegetables include boiling, steaming, pressing, sauteing (both waterless and with oil), and pickling. A variety of natural seasonings, including miso, tamari soy sauce, sea salt, and brown rice vinegar or umeboshi vinegar are recommended in vegetable cooking. Vegetables from tropical climates are not recommended for use in the temperate zones, neither are nightshade vegetables such as tomatoes, potatoes and eggplant. Three to five vegetable side dishes can be prepared daily to ensure adequate variety.

Vegetables in the "Regular Use" column may be eaten daily, while those in the "Occasional Use" column may be eaten once or twice per week on average. In certain cases, especially when a person feels weak or has impaired digestion, it may be necessary to temporarily avoid the intake of raw salad. Instead, dishes such as quickly boiled (blanched) salad, pressed salad, and steamed greens can be eaten daily or often. In normal circumstances, a small amount of high-quality sesame oil can be used about three times per week in sautéing vegetables and other foods; however, when a large volume of high-fat animal foods has been recently consumed, it may be necessary to limit the use of oil for several months until health improves.

Beans

Beans and their products, including tofu, tempeh, natto, and others, comprise about 5 to 10 percent of the standard macrobiotic diet. Any of the following varieties may be selected:

Regular Use
Azuki beans
Black soybeans
Chick-peas (garbanzo
    beans)
Dried tofu (soybean curd
    that has been naturally
    dried)
Fresh tofu
Lentils (green)
Natto (fermented soybeans)
Tempeh (fermented soy-
    beans or combination of
    soybeans and grains)

Occasional Use
Black-eyed peas
Black turtle beans
Great northern beans
Kidney beans
Mung beans
Navy beans
Pinto beans
Soybeans
Split peas
Whole dried
    peas

Beans and bean products are more easily digested when cooked with a small volume of seasonings such as sea salt, miso, or kombu. They may also be prepared with vegetables, chestnuts, dried apples, or raisins, and occasionally sweetened with grain sweeteners like barley malt and rice honey. Serve them in soups and side dishes, or with grains or sea vegetables.

Beans from the "Regular Use" column can be eaten daily, as can tofu, dried tofu, tempeh, and other bean products. Those in the "Occasional Use" column can be eaten two or three times per month, on average. Beans are more digestible when cooked with kombu.

Sea Vegetables

Sea vegetables provide essential minerals and may be used daily in cooking. Wakame and kombu can be used daily in miso and other soups, in vegetable and bean dishes, or in making condiments. Toasted nori is a good source of iron and is also recommended for daily or regular use. Arame and hijiki make wonderful side dishes and can be included several times per week. Agar-agar can be used from time to time in making a natural jelled dessert known as kanten. Below is a list of sea vegetables used in macrobiotic cooking:

Regular Use (daily)
Kombu
Toasted nori
Wakame

Regular Use (several times per week)
Arame
Hijiki

Optional Use
Agar-agar
Dulse
Irish moss
Mekabu
Sea palm
Other traditionally used sea vegetables

White-meat Fish

Low-fat, white-meat fish can be eaten on occasion to supplement the foods already listed. Amounts eaten can vary, depending upon your needs and desires, but generally, several times per week is sufficient. White-meat varieties that are lowest in fat and most easily digested are recommended for regular use.

Ocean Varieties
Cod
Flounder
Haddock

Freshwater Varieties
Bass
Carp
Catfish

Halibut
Herring
Ocean trout
Perch
Scrod
Shad
Smelt
Sole
Other varieties of white-
    meat ocean fish

Pike
Trout
Whitefish
Other varieties of white-
    meat, freshwater fish

Garnishes are especially important in balancing fish and sea-food. Recommended garnishes for persons in good health include: chopped scallions or parsley, grated raw daikon, ginger, radish, or horseradish, green mustard paste (wasabi), raw salad, and shredded daikon. Among the recommended garnishes for fish, a tablespoonful or two of grated raw daikon radish is preferred. Steamed or boiled fish (as in fish soup) is preferable to broiled, baked, deep-fried, or grilled fish.

Fruit

In most cases, fruit can be enjoyed three or four times per week. Locally grown or temperate climate fruits are preferable, while tropical fruits are not recommended for regular use by people in temperate regions. Below are varieties for consumption in temperate climates:

Regular Use	*To Avoid in a Temperate Climate*
Apples	
Apricots	Banana
Blackberries	Dates
Cantaloupe	Figs
Grapes	Pineapple
Honeydew melon	Other tropical or semitropical fruits
Lemons	

Mulberries
Persimmon
Peaches
Plums
Raisins
Raspberries
Strawberries
Tangerines
Watermelon
Wild berries

When fruit is desired, a small serving of northern fruit cooked with a pinch of sea salt can be eaten. However, if fresh fruit is desired during the summer, a small volume can be eaten with a pinch of sea salt sprinkled on it. A small volume of dried fruit can also be eaten on occasion.

Pickles

Pickles can be eaten frequently as a supplement to main dishes. They stimulate appetite and help digestion. Some varieties—such as pickled daikon, or takuan—can be bought prepackaged in natural food stores. Others—such as quick pickles—can be prepared at home.

Regular Use
Amazake pickles
Brine pickles
Miso pickles
Pressed pickles
Rice bran pickles
Sauerkraut
Takuan pickles
Tamari soy sauce pickles

Avoid (for optimal health)
Dill pickles
Garlic pickles
Herb pickles
Spiced pickles
Vinegar pickles

One tablespoonful of naturally processed, non-spicy pickles can be eaten daily. If pickles have a strong salty flavor, rinse them quickly under cold water before eating.

Seeds and Nuts

Seeds and nuts can be eaten from time to time as snacks and garnishes. They can be roasted with or without sea salt, sweetened with barley or rice malt, or seasoned with tamari soy sauce. Seeds and nuts can be ground into butter, shaved and served as a topping or garnish, or used as an ingredient in various dishes, including dessert. Below are varieties that can be used:

Regular Use	*Infrequent Use*
Almonds	Brazil nuts
Black and white sesame seeds	Cashews
Chestnuts	Macadamia nuts
Filberts	Others
Peanuts	
Pecans	
Pine nuts	
Pumpkin seeds	
Small Spanish nuts	
Squash seeds	
Sunflower seeds	
Walnuts	

With the exception of chestnuts, nuts are high in oils and fats. Therefore, it is better to avoid eating them in large quantities. Chestnuts, however, can be used regularly to add a naturally sweet taste to brown rice and other dishes. Up to a cup and a half of lightly roasted, unsalted seeds can be eaten per week. Sunflower seeds are best eaten during the summer.

Snacks

A variety of natural snacks may be enjoyed from time to time, including those made from whole grains, like cookies, bread, puffed cereals, mochi (cakes made of pounded sweet brown rice), rice cakes, rice balls, and homemade sushi. Lightly roasted nuts and seeds may also be eaten as snacks. The following natural snacks are fine for regular use:

> Leftovers (try to eat leftovers by the following day)
> Mochi
> Noodles
> Popcorn (homemade and unbuttered)
> Puffed whole cereal grains
> Rice balls
> Rice cakes
> Seeds
> Sushi (made at home without sugar, seasoning, or MSG)
> Steamed sourdough bread

Snacks that have a drying or tightening effect on the body, such as popcorn, puffed cereals, rice cakes, and baked flour products, are best eaten in moderation. Other snacks can be enjoyed as desired. However, avoid snacking for two and a half to three hours before sleeping.

Condiments

A variety of condiments may be used, some daily and others occasionally. Small amounts can be sprinkled on foods to adjust taste and nutritional value, and to stimulate appetite. They can be used on grains, soups, vegetables, beans, and sometimes desserts. The most frequently used varieties include:

Regular Use

Gomashio (roasted sesame seeds and sea salt)
Tekka (a special condiment made with soybean miso, sesame oil, burdock, lotus root, carrots, and ginger)
Green nori flakes
Sea vegetable powders (with or without roasted sesame seeds)
Umeboshi (salty, pickled plums)

Occasional Use

Cooked miso with scallions or onions
Cooked nori condiment
Roasted and chopped shiso (pickled beefsteak plant leaves)
Roasted sesame seeds
Shio kombu (kombu cooked with tamari soy sauce and water)
Umeboshi or brown rice vinegar

"Regular Use" condiments can be kept on the table and added to whole grain and other dishes as desired. Gomashio and roasted sea vegetable powders can be sprinkled on dishes as you would salt and pepper. About one teaspoonful of these sprinkled condiments can be used daily. Tekka is a stronger condiment and is best used moderately, about a teaspoonful or so per week, on average. Two or three umeboshi plums can be eaten per week along with grains or other dishes. "Occasional Use" condiments can be used about two or three times per week if desired for variety. Condiments that include sea salt are best used in moderation.

Seasonings

It is better to avoid strong spicy seasonings such as curry, hot pepper, and others, and to use those which are naturally processed from vegetable products or natural sea salt, and which have been used as a part of traditional diets. A list of seasonings recommended in the standard macrobiotic diet is presented below:

Regular Use
Miso (fermented soybean and grain paste, i.e., rice, barley, soybean, sesame, and other misos)
Soy sauce
Tamari soy sauce (fermented soybean and grain sauce)
Unrefined sea salt

Occasional Use
Brown rice and umeboshi vinegar
Garlic
Grated daikon, radish, and ginger
Lemon
Mirin (fermented sweet brown rice liquid)
Sesame and corn oil
Umeboshi plum paste
Other traditional natural seasonings

Avoid (for optimal health)
Commercial seasonings
Irradiated spices and herbs
Stimulant and aromatic spices and herbs

In general, use seasonings in moderation. Dishes should have a mild, not salty, flavor. A moderate amount of "Regular Use" seasonings can be used daily in cooking; those in the "Occasional Use" column can be used several times per week for variety. Mirin, which contains a small amount of alcohol, is best avoided temporarily by those seeking to improve their health. Raw garlic is best avoided.

Sweets

The naturally sweet flavor or cooked vegetables can be featured daily for optimal health. Include one or several of the vegetables listed below:

Cabbage	Parsnips
Carrots	Pumpkin
Daikon	Squash
Onions	Sweet vegetable drink or jam

In addition, a small amount of concentrated sweeteners made from whole cereal grains may be included when desired. Dried chestnuts, which also impart a sweet flavor, may also be included on occasion, along with occasional apple juice or cider. Additional natural sweeteners include:

Amazake	Chestnuts (cooked)
Barley malt	Hot apple cider
Brown rice syrup	Hot apple juice

The best sweets are those derived from the complex carbohydrates in whole grains and naturally sweet vegetables, and foods such as chestnuts. Naturally sweet vegetables can be included in various dishes on a daily basis. In addition, sweet vegetable drink can also be used daily or often to relieve the craving for sweets. A small amount of concentrated sweeteners, including grain syrups, amazake, and apple juice, can be used on occasion to relieve the craving for sweets.

Beverages

A variety of beverages may be consumed daily or occasionally. Amounts can vary according to weather conditions and each person's needs. The beverages listed below can be used to comfortably satisfy the desire for liquid.

Regular Use
Bancha stem tea
Bancha twig tea (kukicha)
High-quality natural well water
Natural spring water (suitable for daily use)
Roasted brown rice or barley tea

Occasional Use
Dandelion tea
Freshly squeezed carrot juice (if desired, about two cups per week)
Grain coffee (100 percent roasted cereal grains)
Kombu tea
Sweet vegetable broth
Umeboshi tea

Infrequent Use
Beer (natural quality)
Green leaf tea
Green magma (barley green juice)
Northern climate fruit juice
Sake (fermented rice wine, without chemicals or sugar)
Soymilk
Vegetable juice
Wine (natural quality)

Avoid (for optimal health)
Aromatic herbal teas
Chemically colored tea
Chemically processed beverages
Coffee
Cold or iced drinks
Distilled water
Hard liquor
Mineral water and all bubbling waters
Stimulant beverages
Sugared drinks
Tap water
Tropical fruit juices

Beverages in the "Regular Use" column can be enjoyed on a daily basis, while those in the "Occasional Use" column can be enjoyed two or three times per week. Those suggested for infrequent use are best used only on occasion by those in good general health.

Proper Cooking

Macrobiotic cooking is quick and simple once a few basic techniques—how to use a pressure cooker, wash and cut vegetables, and how to plan menus to ensure adequate taste and variety—are mastered. Before you learn the basics, however, it is easy to make mistakes. This is especially true when getting started, since many of the foods and cooking methods are new and unfamiliar. However, you will develop proficiency in this skill—as in any other—once you become familiar with the ingredients and methods used in macrobiotic cooking.

Recipes and cookbooks are, of course, helpful, but the best way to learn about macrobiotic cooking is to attend classes where you can actually see the foods prepared and can taste them. Most introductory macrobiotic cooking classes are presented in a series of six to eight sessions, and will show you how to do important things like wash and soak foods, cut vegetables, puréed miso for soup, and combine ingredients in complete meals. Advice on menu planning, setting up your kitchen, and shopping for natural foods is usually provided.

Weekly dinners, which many macrobiotic centers sponsor, are also helpful, as they offer you the chance to see and taste a balanced meal and to talk to other people about macrobiotics in a relaxed and supportive setting. Some programs, such as the Macrobiotic Way to Health Seminar presented by the Kushi Institute in the Berkshires, offer a combination of meals and hands-on cooking training. Programs that offer hands-on guidance are the best for learning to cook properly.

Way of Life Suggestions

Together with eating well, there are a number of practices that complement a balanced natural diet and enhance the recovery of health and spirit. Keeping physically active, developing a positive outlook, and using natural cooking utensils, fabrics, and materials in the home are especially recommended. In the past, people lived more closely with nature and ate a more balanced natural diet. With each generation, we have gotten further from our roots in nature, and have experienced a corresponding increase in cancer, heart disease, and other chronic conditions. These suggestions complement the macrobiotic diet and can help everyone enjoy more satisfying and harmonious living.

• Live each day happily without being preoccupied with your health; try to keep mentally and physically active.

• View everything and everyone you meet with gratitude; in particular, offer thanks before and after each meal.

• Chew your food at least fifty times per mouthful, or until it becomes liquid. The complex carbohydrates in whole grains, beans, vegetables, and other whole natural foods are digested largely in the mouth through interaction with the enzymes in saliva. Chewing mixes food with saliva and facilitates smooth digestion and efficient absorption of nutrients. Chewing enables us to obtain more nutrients from less food. It also releases the medicinal properties of daily foods and is the key to improving, rather than simply maintaining, our state of health.

• It is best to avoid wearing synthetic or woolen clothing directly on the skin. Wear cotton as much as possible, especially for undergarments. Avoid excessive metallic accessories on the fingers, wrists, or neck. Keep such ornaments simple and graceful.

• To increase circulation, scrub your entire body with a hot, damp towel every morning or every night. If that is not possible, at least do your hands, fingers, feet, and toes.

• Initiate and maintain active correspondence, extending

your best wishes to parents, children, brothers and sisters, teachers, and friends. Keep your personal relationships smooth and happy.

• Avoid taking long hot baths or showers unless you have been consuming too much salt or animal food.

• If your strength permits, walk outside for up to one half hour every day; wear simple clothes. Keep your home in good order, from the kitchen, bathroom, and living rooms to every corner of the house.

• Avoid chemically perfumed cosmetics. To care for your teeth, brush with natural preparations or sea salt.

• In addition to taking a half-hour walk each day, include activities such as scrubbing floors, cleaning, washing clothes, and working in the yard or garden as a part of your daily life. You may also participate in exercise programs such as yoga, martial arts, dance, or sports if your condition permits.

• Avoid using electric cooking devices (ovens and ranges) or microwave ovens. Convert to gas or wood-stove cooking at the earliest opportunity.

• It is best to minimize the use of color television and computer display terminals. Laboratory studies suggest that electromagnetic fields can interfere with DNA and stimulate chemicals in cells that are linked to cancer. A background paper issued in 1989 by the Congressional Office of Technology Assessment stated, "It is now clear that low frequency electromagnetic fields can interact with individual cells and organs to produce biological changes."

• Place large green plants in your house to freshen and enrich the oxygen content of the air in your home. Houseplants can cut indoor air pollution. According to the Environmental Protection Agency, the air inside closed-ventilation offices can be from two to five times more polluted than outside air. In a recent study of nineteen ordinary plants, NASA researchers found that the plants helped remove three of the most common toxic chemicals from the air, including benzene, formaldehyde, and trichloroethylene.

• Sing a happy song every day in order to activate your breathing and energy flow and elevate your spirits.

• Take an active role in creating your health. As we gain a better understanding of the way that diet and lifestyle influence health and sickness, we are in a better position to make healthful changes in our lives. We shift from a passive to an active role in creating health. The responsibility for making positive changes is up to each of us. No one can take that responsibility for us. We are the ones who must initiate healthful changes and sustain them from day to day.

The Spiral of Healing

Your physical condition becomes cleaner and your memory clearer as you continue to eat macrobiotically. One year of macrobiotic eating changes your condition by seven years. Your body becomes younger, cleansed of the excesses of previous dietary habits. Mental and emotional disturbances are cleared from your memory in the same one to seven ratio. Past eating of meat, sugar, dairy, drugs, chemicals and other nonessential foods directly affects our physical condition. This in turn influences our experiences and our interpretation and memories of them. If, in the past, you had problems in a relationship while eating badly, the impressions translated and processed by your consciousness were influenced by the condition of your blood and brain cells. The nature of our experiences and memories reflect the state of our health.

Eating macrobiotically heals your condition and changes your orientation toward life. You begin to see things with a different perspective. As healing continues on deeper, more subtle levels, events in your past, stored as memories, surface and disappear in the same way that past physical conditions are discharged. It takes about seven years of living macrobiotically to completely reestablish your condition. The rate is dependent, of course, on your understanding and application.

Some people experience difficulties around the time of their seventh year of macrobiotics. They have returned, in memory and condition, to infancy and may begin to crave the foods, like milk and sugar, that they ate as babies. However, they risk negating the years of healing that they have accomplished if they give in to these desires. After passing through this infancy period, we return further into the past, and begin to reestablish the 3.2 billion years of biological evolution we experienced in our mother's womb. Major constitutional changes begin after seven years of macrobiotics. Of course, our constitution is affected before this time, but to a lesser degree.

We perceive a tree visually. We see form, height, color, and so forth in three dimensions. In the Orient, this is called *So*, meaning appearance or shape. In diagnosis, So is expressed as our observation of physiognomy. The Japanese name for this is *Nin-So*. We also perceive images with the mind in a manner more refined than with the eyes. This takes place on the level of memory or image, and can extend over vast distances of time and space. In the invisible, vibrational world we cannot measure things by weight or volume. Physical senses are inadequate in this realm. That is why modern science cannot recognize the spiritual world and why many people do not believe it exists. When our perceptions are clouded by poor eating, our sensitivity does not develop, and so we limit ourselves to the narrow world of physical perception. Although everyone is influenced by more subtle energies, if our condition is not sensitive we have no awareness of them and cannot react to them consciously.

Weight is yang, volume yin. In the physical world, weight is the most accurate form of measure. The spiritual world is measured in terms of time and space. Space is gauged by the distance your image or memory travels. It may be a thousand or a million miles. In comparison to time, space is yin and less stable, and therefore more difficult to measure. For example, if speed is fast, distance shortens. If speed diminishes, space lengthens. Time also changes, but fluctuates less and is thus a more reliable form of measurement. The spiritual world is also reckoned by time.

In the context of time, there is a one to seven ratio between the physical and spiritual worlds. Events change at a rate seven times faster in the spiritual world than in the physical world. If you eat macrobiotically for one year, making your physical condition better and better, you change your vibrational body at a rate that is seven times greater.

If you had pneumonia twenty-one years ago, you repeat this experience after about three years of macrobiotic eating. You may experience similar symptoms, coughing or a fever, for instance, that continue for several days and then suddenly disappear. Deep within, the sickness is being released and is now surfacing and being discharged. In the same way, past experiences and memories start to emerge. It is important that you understand the mechanisms at work and are prepared for these occurrences, rather than becoming discouraged as past problems resurface just as real progress is being made. As you relive past experiences coming from deep within, you perceive them in a different light. You are able to put past experiences into perspective, understand what caused them, perceive their significance, learn their lessons, and then let go of them.

Back along the Spiral

Purification of your embryonic period begins after seven years of macrobiotics. Your constitution also starts to heal. Your thinking changes. Your thoughts turn to your parents and then beyond. You remember the time when you were the foods your parents ate. Later, you regain memories of the animal and the vegetable world, and become aware of your kinship with these stages of life. You are able to see and understand the universe from their vantage point. Every level of life has a unique consciousness and you make contact with each as you retrace the steps of your origin to infinity.

Many vegetarians refrain from eating meat for sentimental or sensory reasons. They see the suffering of animals, or are repelled by the sight and taste of meat and conclude this is immoral. Their actions are correct although their view is limited, and their reasons for acting incomplete. Without understanding the order of the universe, we are not free to act flexibly under any circumstances. The macrobiotic approach is different. From an evolutionary standpoint, we know that animal food is not the proper food for humanity. It does not impart breadth of vision nor foster the development of refined human consciousness. Our motives are based on an understanding of the relationship between food and consciousness.

The elemental world of air, soil, and minerals opens to you as your memory continues to clear. Your kinship with nature can be reestablished. You come to realize that the rocks are speaking to you, the soil whispering its truth, the water singing a song, the wind consoling you, and the stars revealing their secrets. This is not perceived from a sentimental level, nor is it an intellectual or conceptual exercise. It is rather an actual experience, a direct contact with life. You are beginning to communicate with the universe.

The next memory you regain is that of the preatomic world. You begin to see that all things have infinite depth. You understand the world of electrons and protons and realize your existence in and your link with this realm. Life does not stop at the atomic or preatomic level, but rather extends to infinity in all directions. As your healing continues, so does your sensitivity to the existence of energy and vibrations. You see that life is not limited to the narrow parameters of the physical senses. You are spirit, thought, and image. Your physical entity is but a fraction of your total being. You realize that life is limited only by the scope of your awareness and potential circumscribed solely by the boundaries of your imagination. You begin to know your future in the spiritual world. You perceive the meaning of soul as a reality. You view life from a different, a wider, more comprehensive angle that continues to increase until you embrace infinity itself.

As we regain health, we recognize that plants have consciousness, emotions, and wills, and sense their spiritual existence and meaning. Each reflection of life, we realize, is a manifestation of the one great spirit or soul from which all things appear, by which all are sustained, and to which all return. Due to chaotic eating, our thinking has dulled and narrowed. We categorize and isolate life. We judge and value things independently of their relation to the continuous flow and connectedness of existence. We see a tree and instantly fit it into a preconceived and limited set of labels. We generally have no awareness of a tree on the spiritual level, on the conscious level or as a possible entity to communicate and feel kinship with. In this way, we limit our participation in life.

Gradually we reconstruct our existence back along the seven-orbited spiral of materialization. We begin to use the knowledge of these various levels to put our own life in order. The reasons for and solutions to nagging problems become clear. We understand why things happen to us in the way they do and why we continue to attract certain situations. We can use this knowledge to help clear up the present and to create the future. The next stage we contact is the realm of polarization, of differentiation, of yin and yang. All things, including our own life, are the expressions of these two primary forces of the universe. We are now in a position to know the fundamental pattern of life and to change circumstances to produce the results we want. Understanding at this point is very refined. We have penetrated to the basis of existence. The so-called secrets of the universe are known to us.

As our condition continues to improve, we begin to know the oneness of life; all manifestations, we realize, are nothing but differentiated forms of the infinite universe, or God. Human beings, plants and animals, the elemental and preatomic worlds, and the various other realms extending back along the spiral of creation and forward along the spiral of spiritualization are merely representations of the one force that permeates, that gives birth to, sustains, and receives all phenomena. Our understanding of these things will progress beyond the intellectual stage. We know them intuitively without having to play with concepts or philosophies. Perception comes from the center of our being. This is true wisdom. We begin to see that there is never any reason to complain about or resist the things that happen to us. Supreme happiness is within us, always.

The space you are aware of becomes progressively larger while the concept of time grows shorter as your memory proceeds back toward infinity. Eating macrobiotically for seven years will establish your physical condition, but to purify your memory takes seven times seven years of proper eating. Then, you are capable of achieving the universal level of consciousness. However, do not think that someone beginning macrobiotics at the age of fifty will not be able to reach this stage of human development. Humanity's natural life-span is much longer than we realize. Remember that death is an act of will. The seven levels of death are: death by sickness; death by accident; sentimental suicide; psychological suicide; ideological death; natural death; and spiritual death. We die only by our ignorance and our will. People choose the manner and time of their death. There is no reason to die at seventy or eighty years of age. If you want to live longer, you can do so with your understanding of the principles of macrobiotics.

You can accelerate this forty-nine-year developmental period in several ways. First, keep busy. Make full use of each day. Activity shortens our days; inactivity makes them tedious and long. Self-reflection is another aid to development. By understanding the causes of the things that happen to us, we can change our condition so that nagging problems will vanish. People sometimes experience similar circumstances no matter how frequently or drastically they alter exterior conditions. New jobs, new friends, a new home in a new city often do not remedy the mistakes that trouble us. We must turn inward, accept responsibility for all that happens to us and then reflect on what it is in our daily lives that causes the same problems to appear no matter how often superficial conditions change.

As your memory clears, as the past and future become perceptible to you, your judgment will sharpen and your rate of development quicken. If yesterday you ate something salty and it made you think, feel, and act tight, then you will use your judgment to avoid the same mistake. Of course, you will also be able to utilize lessons that are not so recent. Experiences that have occurred in this and past human lives, together with experiences that have taken place on the other levels of existence, are available for your use. Connections will be made between past experiences and tomorrow's possibilities. You will think, "If I do this today, perhaps tomorrow I will lack energy," and the thought will be based on memory.

If your memory is limited to this life or extends only to your human existence, if you cannot use the understanding of the plant and the elemental worlds, along with an understanding of the other levels of existence from which you have come, your potential will be limited. In this case, behavior is not based on conscious awareness but rather on mechanical responses or narrow egocentric motives. If we do something from an emotional, sensory, or intellectual standpoint, without considering the total view of life, the results are the opposite of those intended. Our civilization is built on a foundation of limited perception rather than from the wisdom of a large view. We think and act as if still believing the universe revolves around us. The price we pay for such narrow vision is becoming increasingly apparent. If we pollute our water, air, and soil in an attempt to extract a quick profit, we betray a lack of memory of our own experiences as water, air, and earth. We isolate ourselves from the continuous flow of life. Few people suspect that they are the cause of their own dissatisfaction. Happiness correlates directly to the degree to which we understand life.

The Scope of Macrobiotic Healing

The establishment of physical health is only the first stage in the process of healing. Longevity and freedom from sickness are the natural result of living in harmony with nature and come from practicing the macrobiotic way of life. The second aspect of macrobiotic healing involves developing consciousness and spirituality. Why is food important for developing spirituality? In order to understand this, let us consider a simple analogy.

Suppose we have a television set. In order for the television to work, we must have electricity. Then the various tubes start to receive energy and the television is ready to receive waves from long distances. We can adjust the charge of electricity, its degree and frequency, by adjusting the dials of the set. If the set is built with old-fashioned tubes and wires, meaning that it is less refined than the machines in use today, then it may only be able to receive local stations. If the set is made with more refined, state-of-the-art components, however, it will be able to receive stations from far away and interpret the waves into images and sound. In our bodies, energy is supplied by food. Food charges the entire body with energy. The kind of food determines the kind of energy that each of our cells receives.

Vibrations from the universe are channelled through the nervous system, which is constructed in the form of a spiral. The center of that spiral is the midbrain. This center is very yang. By the strength of the midbrain we can attract various wavelengths, some from short, others from long distances. Our sensory receptors also attract vibrations, but the midbrain has the strongest attracting power, and processes vibrations from the greatest distances. Our eyes can detect vibrations from thousands of light years away, but our brains are capable of receiving even more distant frequencies.

What decides how much vibration we are able to attract? Day to day we change this receiving, interpreting ability. Each of our millions of cells is a spiral. The center of every cell is similar to the midbrain. It attracts vibrations in a similar way. After you receive vibrations, you naturally discharge them. Waves with lower frequencies and longer wavelengths create our bodily activity. Higher frequency, shorter waves create our thoughts, images, and dream. Our spirituality is determined by the degree to which our cells are charged with energy; for example whether they receive short or long waves, high or low frequencies, and how many kinds of waves they are able to receive and process.

Each cell is spirited. In the macrobiotic definition, "spirited" means to be alive and fully charged with energy. If we are able to attract vibrations from far away as well as those nearby, low and high frequencies, and those with longer wavelengths and those with shorter wavelengths, then naturally our world is not small. We can cope with the small relative world and also the far-away world. Spiritual understanding depends on this charge, and this depends on the health of the spiral within each cell, along with the health of the large spiral that makes up the nervous system as a whole. If we eat strong yin foods, such as sugar, spices, or alcohol, our spirals become overexpanded and we cannot catch short waves. We lose our high spirit. When we eat meat, our charge becomes overactive, not refined, and we receive and interpret chaotically.

Through macrobiotics, not only can we secure health, but we can become highly spiritual. Many people make the mistake of thinking that in order to develop spiritually, we need to concentrate on the mind or consciousness while ignoring the condition of the body. However, being a highly developed spiritual person means that we are a highly charged person. When you eat the proper food, you become more highly charged. Our physical condition is equal to our spiritual condition.

When you meet someone you have an impression; he is very nice, honest, or straightforward. That is, you are seeing him physically. But you are also understanding that person spiritually through his expression. Actually we are doing physical and spiritual things equally. Yet, many people separate the spiritual and physical worlds. This is a great mistake that prevents us from reaching a highly developed state.

From our meridians our body charge is distributed to all our cells and body tissues. They all receive energy and vibration. We can transfer these vibrations to others through massage, palm healing, and positive thoughts. If our body is highly charged and spiritual, so that we easily receive high frequencies, we can also send vibrations across distances for the purpose of healing. We can also use words. By talking, discussing, we can change ideas and personalities. Higher levels of communication take place in the form of thought. At this level we do not need to use our senses. This takes place when we use prayer for certain things.

This can work not only for one person, but for a group. When you talk to ten people, or to a hundred people, you move their minds and they change. That is, you use words, which convey the vibrations of thought, to change their personalities. You are like a television station dispatching a message to millions of viewers. You can also send prayers or images to the whole world. Of course, some will not catch them because their receivers are not healthy. But some, who have refined receivers, can receive and interpret these vibrations.

Plants, rocks, soil, and other natural phenomena are also spiral forms and are also charged with energy. If you are healthy, you become sensitive to their energies and are able to communicate with and understand them. Moreover, if your condition is clear and refined, when day changes into night, when the atmosphere and temperature change, you can catch the motion of the constellations and can see and feel how this world is going.

When we eat bad food, a variety of shaky vibrations are produced and our receiver does not work properly. Meditation and breath control help us gain sensitivity to more refined vibrations, just like adjusting the dial on a television set. But among spiritual methods, the way of eating is the highest. Without eating properly, our cells will not be highly charged, and we cannot be a really spiritual person. The macrobiotic way of eating can help everyone become highly spiritualized.

Achieving Our Fullest Potential

A diet of whole grains and vegetables enables us to achieve the maximum scope of biological development. From the primordial gaseous state of the earth about 3.2 billion years ago, life developed in two directions: toward the yin vegetable kingdom and toward the yang animal kingdom. On the scale of animal evolution, life progressed from the stage of primitive single-cell forms (1) through to invertebrates (2), vertebrates, including fish (3), amphibians (4), reptiles and birds (5), mammals (6), and human beings (7). On the vegetable scale, life developed in a parallel way from primitive single-cell forms (1), to primitive water mosses (2), seaweeds (3), land mosses (4), ancient plants (5), modern plants (6) and ultimately, to herb plants, including cereal grains (7).

While in the womb, we are nourished entirely by animal

food provided by our mother's bloodstream. After birth, we are nourished by more yin animal food in the form of mother's milk. When teeth come in, and we stand erect, our nourishment should then come from the world of plants, with whole cereal grains as main foods. If we wish to include some animal food in our diet, it is best to choose the more primitive forms. When we eat mammals as our main foods, we are transforming them into ourselves. However, this transformation works both ways and we also become like mammals; we degenerate and lose our humanity. When we eat fish we are also transforming it into ourselves, but because fish is further back on the evolutionary scale, the person who eats it retains a much larger biological scope than the person who eats land animals.

If we eat sea vegetables, we go beyond the animal kingdom and start to understand the world of vegetables. If we eat on the fifth, sixth, and seventh stages of the vegetable kingdom, our biological scope covers about 6.4 billion years. In other words, we go back along the entire 3.2 billion year course of animal evolution and out along the 3.2 billion year course of vegetable evolution, ending in the cereal plants. This scope is about 128 times greater than if we eat animal food, which in terms of evolution, goes back only about fifty million years.

By eating cereal grains as main foods, in addition to fresh local vegetables, beans, sea vegetables, and other regional supplementary foods, our consciousness, or breadth of vision, becomes 128 times more developed. When people who eat these different ways meet, they cannot understand each other because their view of life is so different. The person who eats farther back can embrace and understand the difference, but the other cannot. Their consciousness is totally different. People who depend mainly on animal foods are limiting their scope of vision. They tend to be confined to the sensory realm.

Unless something can be quantified or measured with the senses, such as is done with modern science, they do not believe it to be real. But beyond the senses are realms thousands of times greater. Of course, we can continue to develop science. But science should not become the leading tool for mankind. Rather it should serve the broader human capacities of intuition and insight.

However, there is a danger inherent in the potential for achieving the fullest scope of biological development. When a bird eats fruit, it does not eat the seeds, and the seeds can sprout and give rise to a new generation of plants. When we eat grains, we are eating the seeds and fruits together, or the beginning and end of plant life. This is the most naturally balanced way of eating on earth, but also contains within it the possibility of self-extinction. Thus, if we exercise our appetite without limit, we risk becoming extinct because food will no longer be available. Therefore we need self-control and moderation. All ethics begin from that point. Social morality is small by comparison because it is based on the assumption that everyone is living. If the supply of grains runs out, then humanity cannot continue on this planet. Few people are aware of this biological code of ethics. In the biological world, there is an unspoken code based on common sense, and that is simply not to overeat. It is important to be grateful for what we eat and to chew thoroughly, not only for health but to use our food for maximum efficiency. By eating a small volume and chewing well, we can maintain this biological code and also secure health.

Future Adaptations

Eating grains and vegetables, and cooking properly, can help humanity pass through climatic changes, including periods of global cooling and global warming. Aside from disruptions caused by modern industry and civilization, these periods arise because of natural, cosmic cycles, including the movement of the solar system around the center of the Milky Way. The solar system revolves around the galactic center in a cycle lasting approximately 200 million years. We can divide this cycle into four sections, each lasting for about 50 million years. During part of the cycle, the solar system moves closer to galactic center and contracts, causing temperatures on earth and the other planets to rise. During the opposite part of the cycle, the solar system moves further from the center of the galaxy and expands, and average temperatures decrease. This cycle is like a vast galactic year, which like the solar year, can be divided into four seasons.

About 100 million years ago, the earth was in the middle of galactic summer. At that time, life took the form of giant reptiles and large, expanded plants. As the earth entered galactic autumn, temperatures became cooler and these expanded life forms could not continue. Thus the dinosaurs became extinct and were replaced by mammals, and ancient plants gave way to more compact, modern species. Eventually, cooler temperatures gave rise to cereal grains, the most compact form of plant life. Eating this newer form of food, mammals and apes evolved toward homo sapiens. About a million years ago, the earth approached the peak of galactic winter and the cycle of Ice Ages began. Before that, our ancestors ate grains and other plant foods raw. In order to adapt to the Ice Ages, our ancestors learned how to use fire and salt in cooking. These developments led to the development of culture and civilization, including human consciousness and spirituality.

Four Ice Ages have occurred since the cycle of glaciation began one million years ago. Another Ice Age will take place in the future. In order to survive under conditions such as these, our descendents will need knowledge of yin and yang and proper cooking. In this way humanity can continue without being destroyed by severe cold. Through the application of fire, salt, oil, and pressure, and the selection of foods that help us to harmonize with environmental conditions, humanity can live comfortably through the coming Ice Age, which in my estimate, will arrive in about 150,000 years. Then, when the earth enters galactic spring, and warmer weather eventually comes, humanity can change its cooking by applying fewer yang factors. By knowing yin and yang, humanity can gain the ability to survive and prosper throughout the ages.

The expansion and contraction of the solar system resulting from its motion around the center of the galaxy occurs within a much larger movement in which the planets gradually spiral in toward the sun. The solar system is not, as is presently assumed, a series of concentric circles in which the planets take fixed orbits around the sun. It is a vast logarithmic spiral. This spiral begins at the periphery and moves toward the center. The planets slowly migrate from the periphery to the center, and eventually melt into the sun. In the far distant future, the earth will begin to approach the present orbit of Venus; at that time, temperatures on earth will be too hot to support life. At the same time, Mars will approach the present orbit of the earth and primitive vegetation may start to appear. Eventually it may become ready to support human life. At that time, perhaps about 400 million years from now, our descendants will be able to carry the understanding of yin and yang, food selection, and proper cooking to Mars and start to build a new civilization.

A similar migration may have occurred in the remote past. Civilizations may have developed long ago on Venus, but as this planet came closer to the sun, approaching its present orbit, it became too hot to support life and the people living there may have migrated to earth, bringing with them knowledge of cereal grains, fire, and cooking. This pattern of migration may continue until all of the outer planets are inhabited. In the case of Jupiter and the planets beyond it, it will take a long time before they are ready to support human life. The practice of macrobiotics and the understanding of yin and yang can enable humanity to enjoy practically unlimited security and continue as long as the solar system exists. On an individual level, the practice of macrobiotics leads to a feeling of inner peace and security within the endless order of change.

A New Species of Humanity

At the present time, applying the principles of macrobiotics means that we make cereal grains the central part of our diets. However, macrobiotics is not limited to cereal grains, miso, or tamari soy sauce. Foods such as these are the best items that we now use for our health and adaptation. However, the meaning of macrobiotics is that as the outer environment changes, we change our food.

When we were in the mother's womb, we were eating animal food, in the form of thick liquid (mother's blood). After birth, we are nourished by mother's milk, which is still liquid but lighter than blood. When we eat food, we take it in liquid form through chewing. This food, in comparison with mother's milk and blood, is very light. Then, together with the liquid form of food we also take in air. When more primitive forms of life eat, they eat more than their body weight. Birds, for example, eat plenty. As biological evolution progresses, species eat less physical food and more air and vibration, including energy from the sun, stars, and celestial bodies. If we eat plenty of physical food, we receive less vibration because we are continually discharging excess from our food. If we eat small amounts, we receive a more intense charge of vibration. When we fast, for example, we sometimes have wonderful insights. Eating through the nervous system and eating through the digestive system are complementary and antagonistic. The more solid food we eat, the less air we receive. Ideally, our intake of food should be just enough to charge us and allow us to receive the maximum amount of vibration.

As we get older, our need for physical food becomes less. Your charge becomes greater and you are able to live almost anywhere; in hot or cold weather, or high in the mountains or on the plains. In Japan, there are legends of highly developed spiritual people who lived in the mountains. They were referred to as *Sen-Nin*, or "mountain men." They ate little and lived long lives free from sickness or unhappiness. Their bodies were highly energized and they were not concerned much with the material world. There is a relationship between the volume of food we eat and the volume of material things we are attracted to. The person who eats less is less attached to material things. He or she is more easily satisfied. Although Sen-Nin were few in number, everyone has the potential to achieve the same degree of spiritual development. A high degree of spirituality can become everyone's daily reality as they learn how to change themselves through the understanding of yin and yang. Humanity can thus evolve toward a totally new species, homo spiritus, through the practice of macrobiotics.

As humanity becomes more spiritually developed, our primary food will become vibration which we can use to create our energy and Ki flow, in addition to our muscles, skin, bones, and physical form. At this stage, people will be able to materialize their bodies and life directly from the vibrational world. Whatever they think, they will be able to materialize, or bring forth in themselves and others. If someone with this ability wishes to obtain something, he or she can obtain it by using vibration and applying yin and yang. When these abilities become widespread, humanity will no longer need scientific technology. Moreover, as humanity develops spiritual qualities, people will be able to determine how long they want to live, and will gain freedom from the cycle of life and death. People will be able to attain this freedom naturally, and not through special efforts or training. These abilities will be realized by everyone, and not by just a chosen few.

Today, people are degenerating, biologically, mentally, and spiritually. Many people are fearful, many are developing degenerative diseases, and civilization itself is being threatened by war and environmental destruction. However, through macrobiotics, humanity can change direction and develop into a new species that is not bothered by the negative things that have been experienced in the past. Those who overcome and pass through the modern crisis can emerge as a new race with a new vision. From now on, the real history of humanity is beginning. All history until now has only been the prelude to this beginning; the first chapter in the new history of humanity, or the age of human health, happiness, and freedom, is about to begin.

7
Food as Medicine

We constantly receive energy from heaven and earth. Heaven's yang, downward force and earth's yin, upward force run along a primary channel deep within the body. These forces charge the body and all of its functions, and it is along this central line that seven energy centers, or chakras, arise. Lines of energy, or meridians, radiate outward from this central line toward the surface of the body in the way that the ridges of a pumpkin branch outward from its central core. The meridians charge each of the organs and subdivide into smaller streams that provide energy to each cell.

Heaven and earth do not charge both sides of the body equally; heaven's force is stronger on one side, and earth's force on the other side. So, although both sides of the body appear similar, they actually function in an opposite, yet complementary way. When we walk or run, for example, we put the right foot forward and the left foot backward, and vice versa, in an alternating pattern. As we move our right arm to the front, our left moves to the rear, and vice versa.

How then, can we tell which of these forces is stronger on the left and which is stronger on the right side of the body? Most people use their right hand for active, outward, and expansive movements, and their left for supportive, stabilizing, or contractive movements. When writing, for example, the right hand moves outward as the pen glides across the page, while the left counterbalances by keeping still and applying pressure to the paper. When throwing a ball, the right arm thrusts forward away from the body, while the left moves in the opposite direction toward the rear. The right hand is used for throwing, and the left for catching and receiving. When swinging a bat, most people use their right arm to push the bat forward, and the left to pull in the opposite direction. These basic tendencies also appear among left-handed people. When a left-handed person uses a pen or pencil, for example, they often do so by curling the left wrist inward in the form of a contracting spiral as they write.

Another clue is found in the structure of the large intestine. The large intestine moves up the right, across the middle, and down the left side of the body. At the opposite end of the body, the right brain produces artistic, intuitive thinking (yin), while the left brain generates analytical or rational thinking (yang). As we can see, earth's rising energy predominates on the right side of the body, and heaven's downward, stabilizing force is stronger on the left.

Daily foods can also be understood in terms of these primary forces. In Chapter 6, we classified foods into three categories: extreme yin, extreme yang, and centrally balanced. Extreme yang foods are strongly charged by heaven's downward force. These extreme "downward" foods include eggs, meat, poultry, shellfish, and red meat or blue skinned fish such as salmon, tuna, and bluefish. Extreme yin foods are strongly charged with earth's rising energy. Strong "upward" foods include sugar, chocolate, spices, tropical fruits, soft drinks, ice cream, nightshade vegetables, and drugs and medications. Centrally balanced foods, including grains, beans, fresh local vegetables, and sea vegetables are neither strongly "upward" nor strongly "downward." Although they receive energy from heaven and earth, on the whole they are more evenly balanced than the extremes indicated above.

Foods from either extreme disrupt the smooth flow of energy in the body. Eating plenty of meat, cheese, chicken, or other foods with strong downward energy blocks or suppresses the flow of earth's upward force on the right side of the body. As the excessive fat and protein contained in these foods accumulate, the organs and blood vessels become hard, tight, and enlarged. These foods produce tension throughout the body.

Energy blockages like these affect not only our physical health and appearance; they also affect our moods and emotions. When upward energy on the right side of the body becomes blocked because of strong "downward" foods, we start to feel impatient and frustrated. We may become irritable and short-tempered, and feel we are being blocked or prevented from doing what we want. If blocked energy continues accumulating, it may burst forth in a sudden, uncontrollable eruption that we call "anger." An outburst of anger, whether expressed physically (yang) or in the form of words (yin), is similar to the eruption of a volcano.

The pancreas is located on the left side of the body where the opposite, downward flow of heaven's force is stronger. Overconsumption of strong yin foods—especially simple sugars—offsets this energy and weakens cells in the pancreas that secrete insulin. Insulin, a yang hormone that lowers blood sugar, is strongly charged with heaven's force. Eating too many strong upward foods can weaken the cells that secrete insulin and dilute that hormone to the point that it lacks the power to lower blood sugar. This condition is known as *diabetes*.

Overconsumption of strong downward foods produces the opposite effect. If the diet contains plenty of cheese, chicken, eggs, and shellfish, downward energy begins to accumulate in the pancreas. Hard fats also build up in the organ, causing tightness and stagnation. These conditions weaken the pancreas' ability to secrete anti-insulin, the hormone that performs a function opposite to that of insulin. Anti-insulin causes the blood sugar level to rise. Normally, both hormones function together to keep the level of blood sugar within a normal range. However, if anti-insulin is deficient, the person may begin to experience chronic low blood sugar, or hypoglycemia. This widespread disorder produces symptoms such as fatigue, depression, and the craving for sweets.

How, then, can we use daily food to restore balance in the internal organs, facial features, and our condition as a whole? The key to this is the understanding of *energetic compatibility*, or knowing how to match the energy in foods with the energy of the organs, meridians, and chakras. For example, foods such as leafy greens, barley, and naturally fermented products reflect earth's upward energy in a moderate way, and promote the smooth flow of upward energy in the body. Eating these items helps restore health and harmony in the ascending colon, liver, gallbladder, right lung, and other organs on the right side of the body that are especially charged by this energy. On the other hand, foods, such as millet, squash, and cabbage are moderately charged with downward energy. Eating them promotes the smooth flow of heaven's force in the body, and helps restore the spleen, pancreas, left lung, descending colon, and other organs on the left side of the body to a healthy condition. Of course, in order to restore balance to any organ or part of the body, it is necessary to avoid extremes and provide the body as a whole with a wide range of energies by including a variety of high-quality natural foods in the diet. Then, within the range of centrally balanced foods, we include those that match the particular organ while restoring harmony to the body as a whole.

In the classification presented below, we list the organs in pairs—with yang, solid or compact organs discussed together with yin, hollow or expanded ones. The organs in each pair complement each other, and function as a complete energy system.

Liver and Gallbladder (Upward or Tree Energy)

The liver and gallbladder are located on the right side of the body, and are charged primarily by earth's rising energy. In the five transformations, they are classified under the stage of upward or tree energy.

Seasonal and Daily Correspondence The liver and gallbladder correspond to springtime and morning, the time of year or day when upward, tree energy is strongest in the atmosphere.

Mental/Emotional Correspondence When energy in the

liver becomes unbalanced, a person has the tendency to feel or express anger. Imbalance in the gallbladder manifests as complaining.

Dietary Adjustments Foods with mildly upward, or expanding energy (tree nature) help energize and restore balance to the liver and gallbladder. Among the grains, barley, a light, expansive grain, is especially charged by earth's rising energy, as is whole wheat. Varieties that are planted in winter and harvested in spring are especially charged with upward energy. Whole barley, hato mugi (pearl barley) or whole wheat berries can be included in your diet several times per week as secondary grains. You can add 15 to 20 percent barley or wheat berries to your brown rice dishes. Barley can be used to make delicious soups, and included in a variety of other dishes. Natural, unyeasted sourdough bread, udon noodles, seitan (wheat-meat), and other products made from whole wheat flour can also be included several times per week, on the average, by those in good health. However, overconsumption of hard, baked flour products can cause tightness in the body that restricts the smooth flow of upward energy.

Natural fermentation, a process in which foods break down and decompose through the action of bacteria, is a product of earth's rising or expansive energy. The energy of naturally fermented foods matches that in the liver and gallbladder. Naturally processed miso made from barley and soybeans is especially good for these organs, as are umeboshi plum, sauerkraut, pickled vegetables—especially light or quick pickles—and naturally processed umeboshi and brown rice vinegar. However, naturally fermented foods are made with sea salt (a strong contracting food that helps balance the expanding energy of fermentation), and are best used in moderate amounts as seasonings or condiments.

Certain vegetables activate the flow of upward energy in the body. Vegetables are nourished by both heaven and earth. Roots grow down below the soil under the influence of heaven's force. Leafy greens branch upward, above the soil. The energy in leafy greens—especially the tops of daikon, carrots, turnips, and dandelion—closely matches the upward energy that nourishes the liver and gallbladder. Leafy green vegetables are best included daily as a part of a balanced macrobiotic diet. Barley miso soup, in which leafy greens are included, is also excellent for the liver and gallbladder.

Interestingly, until modern times, many traditional cooks picked fresh dandelions and other wild greens in the spring and included them in their menus. Spring is the season in which earth's rising energy starts to become active, and is when we naturally seek fresh light dishes to balance the environment. Eating dandelions, chives, scallions, and other fresh greens at this time helps release stagnation in the body caused by previous consumption of more contracted foods during the winter.

Fruits with a naturally sour taste, such as plums and sour apples, can also be used on occasion to release tension and stagnation in the liver and gallbladder. Because of their strong expansive nature, fruits are best cooked with a pinch of sea salt before being eaten. Fire and salt are contracting influences, and counterbalance the strong upward energy in fruits. However, a small volume of fresh fruit grown in the temperate zones may be eaten on occasion by those in good health. A small volume of high-quality natural barley malt may also be used from time to time to release tightness in the body.

Heart and Small Intestine (Active or Fire Energy)

The heart and small intestine are charged by actively expanding fire energy. The heart is located on the primary channel of energy, the central meridian that runs deep within the body and nourishes the chakras, meridians, meridian branches, and cells. The most active charge of energy is found along this channel. The rhythmic pulse of heaven's and earth's forces along the primary channel directly energizes the heart chakra and produces the expansion and contraction of the heart. The small intestine is complementary to the heart. The center of the small intestine, the hara chakra, is situated along the central channel, and actively charged by the energies of heaven and earth that flow along this line.

Seasonal and Daily Correspondence The heart and small intestine correspond to summer and noon, times when active fire energy is predominant in the atmosphere.

Mental/Emotional Correspondence Energy imbalance in the heart results in excessive talking. Weakness in the hara or small intestine as a whole leads to frequent changes of mind and a lack of fortitude or "guts."

Dietary Adjustments Foods with extreme energies are detrimental to the heart and small intestine, and to the circulatory and digestive systems as a whole. Normally the arteries and blood vessels are open and flexible. Eating too many animal foods can cause them to become clogged with deposits of fat and cholesterol. If the blood vessels become narrow and constricted because of these accumulations, blood no longer flows smoothly through them. When this happens in the blood vessels that supply the heart, the result can be a heart attack. When it occurs in the blood vessels that supply the brain, the result may be a stroke. Both conditions are common today because people eat plenty of eggs, cheese, meat, and other fatty animal foods. As you can see, eating foods with extreme contractive energy restricts or suppresses the heart's natural function in distributing blood outward to the body. An overly constricted condition in the heart and circulatory system frequently appears as hardening at the tip of the nose. This condition is usually accompanied by bodily inflexibility and hard, dry skin.

The other major type of heart disease arises because of too many extremely yin foods in the diet. Sugar, alcohol, chocolate, soft drinks, ice cream, and drugs and medications weaken the heart muscle and blood vessels. This can produce a wide variety of conditions including mitral valve prolapse, high blood pressure, enlargement of the heart, and others. An overly expanded condition in the circulatory system appears externally as enlargement or swelling at the tip of the nose, or sometimes as a reddish color—caused by dilation of the capillaries below the skin—on the tip of the nose or face as a whole.

As an example of how overconsumption of strong yin foods or beverages effects the heart, a study published in the February 1989 *New England Journal of Medicine* revealed that long-term overconsumption of alcohol was damaging to the heart and other muscles of the body. In a study of fifty alcoholic men conducted at the University of Barcelona, almost half the subjects had deteriorating muscle strength that was directly related to the total amount of alcohol consumed. Although not mentioned in the study, long-term overconsumption of sugar, chocolate, tropical fruits, soft drinks, and other extremely yin foods or beverages has a similar effect.

Our digestive tract is ideally suited to digesting plant foods. Human intestines are longer than those of carnivores such as lions and tigers. Our long, convoluted intestines provide ample opportunity for animal foods to break down into toxic bacteria and compounds such as ammonia. The toxic by-products generated by the decomposition of animal foods accumulate in the intestines and deplete the stock of beneficial bacteria found there, while the saturated fats in animal foods clog the capillaries in the intestinal villi and diminish their powers of absorption.

Strong expansive foods cause the villi to become chronically dilated, and this also weakens their ability to absorb digested food particles. These conditions can lead to a situation in which someone must continually eat larger amounts of food in order to obtain nutrients. They wind up eating more and using less. The result is overweight combined with nutritional deficiency.

Among the grains and their immediate relatives, corn corresponds to fire energy and restores balance to the heart and small intestine. Corn that is freshly picked in summer is especially beneficial. It can be eaten on the cob (without butter), or used in soups, vegetable, sea vegetable, and a variety of other dishes. Summer vegetables, including cucumber, broad leafy greens such as mustard greens and Chinese cabbage, and other fresh, farm and garden produce, also help dissolve deposits of fat and cholesterol in the circulatory system.

Sea vegetables embody qualities of flexibility and strength that are ideal for toning the heart and circulatory vessels. Their flexibility comes from growing in a watery environment where they gently sway back and forth under the influence of tides and ocean currents. Their strength comes from their high mineral content. When eaten regularly as a part of a balanced diet, sea vegetables such as wakame, kombu, arame, and hijiki impart strength and resilience to the circulatory system as a whole.

Plants from the sea are also good for the intestines. The villi in the small intestines are like single-celled amoeba or primitive sea plants that suck in and absorb nutrients. Sea vegetables, which are more ancient or primitive than land plants, strengthen the villi. Naturally fermented foods also have a primitive nature, due to the bacteria and enzymes they contain. Eating them helps strengthen the beneficial bacteria that inhabit the small intestine. (These bacteria are depleted by sugar, meat, dairy food, and antibiotics.) When used properly, fermented foods such as pickles, sauerkraut, umeboshi plum, and fermented soybean foods like miso and tamari soy sauce are all beneficial to the intestines. Miso soup, in which wakame, kombu, or other sea vegetables are included, is especially good for strengthening the small intestine.

Pancreas, Spleen, and Stomach (Downward or Soil Energy)

The pancreas and spleen have a solid and compact structure and are energized by the downward flow of heaven's force on the left side of the body. The hollow and expanded stomach is complementary to these organs and is also nourished by downward energy on the left side.

Seasonal and Daily Correspondence The spleen, pancreas, and stomach correspond to late summer and afternoon, both times when downward, or soil energy is stronger in the earth's atmosphere.

Mental/Emotional Correspondence Imbalances in spleen and pancreas lead to chronic doubt or suspicion. Disruption in the flow of energy in the stomach frequently manifests as anxiety or worry.

Dietary Adjustments Complex carbohydrates have strong contracting, or downward energy, and harmonize the energy and function of these organs. Good sources of complex carbohydrates include whole grains, beans, naturally sweet vegetables such as cabbage, fall squash, carrots, and onions, sea vegetables, and chestnuts. Complex carbohydrates help the pancreas maintain proper levels of glucose in the blood.

Millet corresponds to soil energy and is especially good for restoring balance in these organs. It can be eaten several times per week. You can cook it together with brown rice in your main grain dish, or combine it with naturally sweet vegetables such as squash or carrots to make delicious soups. Soft millet makes a delicious porridge that is especially nourishing and soothing in the morning. Sweet brown rice also provides a natural sweetness that harmonizes the energy in these organs, and can be included as a special grain from time to time. Sweet brown rice is especially delicious when cooked with dried chestnuts, also a good source of complex carbohydrates. Pounded sweet brown rice, or mochi, is an excellent source of natural sweetness, and can be eaten as a snack.

Naturally sweet vegetables are also good for the energy balance in these organs. The desire for sweetness is natural and instinctive. Everyone is attracted to the sweet flavor to balance the naturally salty bloodstream and because of the body's constant need for energy. Newborn babies, for example, instinctively seek the natural sweetness in mother's milk, and this yin sweetness enables them to grow. However, when choosing foods with sweet flavors, it is important to choose those of the highest quality. If we choose wisely, meaning the high-quality, naturally sweet flavor of whole grains, beans, sweet-tasting vegetables, and other complex carbohydrate foods, we can maintain good health throughout life. If we choose unwisely, meaning the processed, artificially sweet flavor of simple sugar, we risk losing our health. We consider complex carbohydrates "natural" because their sweetness is readily available as is. Whole grains harvested from the field or sweet vegetables taken from the garden require no processing, other than cooking and thorough chewing, to extract their naturally sweet flavor. On the other hand, refined and processed sugars require a great deal of processing to extract their sweetness. Tropical fruits, which also contain simple sugars, are not native to temperate climates, and are available in those regions only because of artificial methods of transportation and refrigeration, in addition to chemically intensive agriculture.

For maximum health and enjoyment, it is important to base each meal around the naturally sweet flavor of whole grains, beans, sweet-tasting vegetables, and other complex carbohydrate foods. The other flavors—sour, bitter, spicy, and salty—are best kept mild and used to contrast and bring forth the naturally sweet flavor of these foods. In macrobiotic cooking, the sour taste is provided by foods such as umeboshi plums, sauerkraut and other pickled vegetables, sour fruits like apples, plums, and occasionally lemon, and naturally fermented umeboshi and brown rice vinegar. The bitter taste is provided by leafy green vegetables such as watercress, parsley, daikon, carrot, turnip, mustard, and other greens, and by condiments and other foods that are lightly roasted. A mild spicy flavor comes from chopped raw scallions, grated raw daikon, and natural mustard or ginger which may be used occasionally. A salty flavor is provided by the moderate use of condiments, seasonings, pickles, and other foods that are naturally processed with sea salt. Again, these supplementary flavors are best kept mild and used to highlight, rather than overwhelm or cover up, the natural sweetness of complex carbohydrates.

Naturally sweet grains and vegetables also restore balance to the stomach and spleen. Chewing is essential, as saliva, a mildly alkaline substance, helps neutralize strong acid in the stomach. Umeboshi plums, which have an alkalizing effect in the body, are especially helpful in rebalancing and strengthening the stomach and digestive organs. They can be used as condiments several times per week or in making ume-sho-kuzu, a traditional home remedy for neutralizing an overacid stomach and strengthening the digestive organs as a whole.

Carbohydrates and Diabetes In the pancreas there are isles. These isles have three different kinds of cells besides tissue cells. One is small, yang; another is a little bigger and more yin; and the other is in-between. The small ones secrete insulin and if the blood sugar is up, this hormone tries to make the sugar level low. The other yin type of cell secretes anti-insulin, making the sugar level go up if it is low. This balance controls the sugar level in the blood. But suppose the two combinations are not working well. In many cases, the small cells start to expand. If the cells secreting insulin do not work properly, the sugar level becomes too high, and the result is diabetes. If the opposite condition arises, meaning that the yin pancreatic cells become tight and constricted, the sugar level stays low, resulting in hypoglycemia.

Overexpansion of the small cells in the pancreas is the result of too many yin foods and drinks. In order to control this condition, we need to limit the intake of extreme yin foods and drinks, especially carbohydrates. Another name for carbohydrates is sugar. Grains such as brown rice are 70 percent sugar, so while we are chewing them they become sweeter and sweeter. The same is true with carrots, squash, and pumpkins. These foods are composed largely of glucose. Other types of sugar include lactose, or milk sugar, sucrose, or cane sugar, and fructose, or fruit sugar. Our bodies need carbohydrates for energy. Among the varieties of carbohydrate, glucose is the most yang form. Sucrose is the most yin. For optimal health, we need to eat a greater volume of polysaccharides and fewer monosaccharides or disaccharides. In polysaccharides, many sugar molecules combine, forming a highly complex structure. In disaccharides, two sugar molecules combine to form a looser, less tightly structured molecule. Monosaccharides are composed of a single molecule of sugar. They are not bound together and exist as separate molecules. Monosaccharides have the most intense sweet flavor.

Drugs, alcohol, and spices—especially hot spices—are more yin or expansive than sugar. One teaspoonful of sugar is very sweet and has a strongly expansive effect on the body. With drugs, a much smaller amount produces a strong effect on the body and mind. Strong spices are also more concentrated than sugar; tiny amounts produce strong yin effects. If we consume these extremes, the yang, compact organs in the body change and start to become expanded. The intestinal juices, saliva, and hormones also change and become strongly acid or yin. Although a general standard exists, everyone's digestive juice has a different composition, as does everyone's blood, saliva, and hormones.

Until recently, as a part of the treatment of diabetes, doctors recommended stopping all sugar, meaning all varieties of carbohydrate, and eating primarily animal protein. This approach mistakenly assumed high blood sugar to be the result of eating too much carbohydrate. Many diabetic patients were told to eat plenty of animal protein. However, diabetes cannot be cured in this way, since protein is more yin than carbohydrate. In order to eat protein, we need salt to make balance. A food such as ham, for example, is very salty, and when someone eats eggs or beef they usually add plenty of salt. Eating plenty of meat, chicken, or eggs cannot help diabetes at all.

Glucose is the most yang form of carbohydrate. To recover from diabetes, yang complex carbohydrates should form the basis of the diet. A person with diabetes also needs a good source of minerals; especially foods such as natural sea salt and sea vegetables. Overall, the person's diet can slightly emphasize yang factors. The person can eat grains with a higher proportion of minerals, which means grains with hard covers or skins, such as yellow millet. Millet is a hard, tiny grain. In addition, vegetables with a higher proportion of glucose, including pumpkin, acorn and butternut squash can be eaten. Sea vegetables provide a good source of minerals, and the yang form of protein in azuki beans helps restore the pancreas to a normal functioning. Roasted sesame oil, which is yang in comparison to unroasted oil, also helps the pancreas return to normal. Hard, leafy vegetables such as carrot and daikon tops, contain plenty of fiber, carbohydrate, and minerals and can also be included as a part of a diet for recovery from diabetes.

It is difficult for persons who develop diabetes during their teenage years to recover completely with diet, although tremendous improvement is possible, including a reduction in the likelihood of related symptoms such as blindness, kidney failure, and heart disease. It is much easier for persons who develop diabetes after age forty to recover. Juvenile diabetes occurs frequently today because children are fed sweets and soda from a young age. Their sugar comes from milk, fruit, honey, and refined sugar. They are eating mono- and disaccharides every day while ignoring foods that contain glucose.

The body stores excess sugar in the liver. This excess can be used for future needs. The liver's storage capacity is about fifty grams. Excess is stored in the form of polysaccharide glucose. When this stored glucose is needed by the body, it is decomposed into a simple form and released by the liver into the bloodstream. In the same way, the main source of sugar in our diets should be polysaccharide glucose. These polysaccharides are gradually decomposed through digestion into di- and monosaccharides. Juvenile diabetics often have large appetites and crave water and oil. In order to meet these cravings, good cooking is especially important.

In a study conducted at the Hospital for Sick Children in Toronto, and published in the August 1992 *New England Journal of Medicine*, drinking cow's milk in infancy was found to be a possible trigger for development of juvenile diabetes. The study suggests that the immune system confuses a type of cow's milk protein, known as bovine serum albumin, with a type of protein found on the surface of the yang, insulin-producing cells in the pancreas. Antibodies made to neutralize the milk protein instead neutralize and destroy the insulin cells.

"If all this holds up, it would be the first autoimmune disease where we have any idea at all about the cause, how it arises and how it is sustained," said Dr. Hans-Michael Dosch, senior author of the study.

Lungs and Large Intestine (Condensed or Metal Energy)

The lungs are densely packed with blood vessels and tiny air sacs known as alveoli. They have a dense, compact structure and are counterbalanced in the body by the large intestine, a long (about 1.5 meters) hollow tube squeezed like an accordion into a tight space. Both organs span the left and right sides of the body, and represent condensed metal energy.

Seasonal and Daily Correspondence The lungs and large intestine correspond to autumn and evening, times when the earth's atmosphere is strongly charged with contracting energy.

Mental/Emotional Correspondence Imbalance in the lungs leads to feelings of sadness or melancholy. Weakness in the large intestine produces the tendency toward indecision, uncertainty, and a loss of clear thinking.

Dietary Adjustments Because of their condensed energy, the lungs and large intestine are particularly sensitive to yang extremes, including meat, eggs, cheese, poultry, and other animal foods. Our long and convoluted digestive tract is perfectly suited to the breakdown and absorption of plant fibers. Energetically, there is a tremendous difference between plant and animal foods. The minerals, proteins, carbohydrates, and fats in plants are highly stable, while the proteins and other nutrients in animal foods are unstable. Whole grains, for example, retain their life energy and nutritive value for hundreds or even thousands of years, and as macrobiotic cooks around the world have discovered, grains, beans, sea vegetables, and other vegetable foods can be stored without refrigeration or artificial preservation. On the other hand, animal foods decompose quickly, and a great deal of effort is required to slow the speed at which they decompose into toxic compounds and bacteria. This unstable character creates numerous problems in the large intestine.

It is now known that the rates of colon cancer are highest among people in the modern, industrialized countries who consume a great deal of meat, poultry, and dairy food, and lowest among people in Asian, African, and Latin American countries where animal food is eaten much less often. Conversely, the rates of colon cancer are highest among people who consume little dietary fiber and lowest among those for whom fiber is a major part of the diet. Interestingly, the relationship between consumption of animal food and consumption of vegetable fiber tends to be complementary and antagonistic. People who eat a great deal of animal food consume less fiber, while those who eat plenty of fiber tend to consume less animal food. In the past, dietary fiber formed a greater part of people's diets worldwide, but as the intake of animal food increased in the twentieth century, consumption of fiber went down. According to some estimates, the intake of fiber is now about one-fifth what it was a hundred years ago, mostly as the result of a steep drop in grain consumption. It was during this time that the rates of colon, breast, and other cancers, heart disease, and other degenerative conditions increased sharply.

Overintake of sugar, chocolate, ice cream, tropical fruits, tomatoes, potatoes, and other nightshade vegetables, drugs and medications, and other yin extremes can cause the intestine to become swollen and loose. In this condition, intestinal contractions may become too weak to move wastes through with regularity, and chronic constipation results. Milk and milk products also contribute to this problem by causing irritation and allergic reactions in the digestive tract. Allergy to cow's milk begins in infancy and takes the form of frequent digestive upsets, irritation, diarrhea, and other problems in the digestive tract that continue throughout life. Milk, milk products, and simple sugars also cause sticky mucus to accumulate in the lungs and large intestine, resulting in a lessening of the capacity to absorb oxygen and discharge carbon dioxide and other waste products. A lack of oxygen in the bloodstream contributes to anemia and stale, unhealthy looking skin.

Among the grains, brown rice corresponds to metal energy and is ideal for restoring health to these organs. Brown rice matures and is harvested in the autumn, a season of downward or condensed energy (metal) in the atmosphere that matches the energy of the lungs and large intestine. Brown rice also has an ideal balance between minerals, proteins, and carbohydrates, making it suitable for use as a principal grain throughout the year. Brown rice is also easy and delicious to eat in its whole form. There is no need to crush it into flour or process it in some way. Moreover, the fiber in rice bran (contained in the outer coat of brown rice) has been found to be effective in reducing cholesterol. Recent studies conducted by the U.S. Department of Agriculture found that a diet including 10 percent dietary fiber from rice bran reduces cholesterol by more than 15 percent. Other whole grains also contain fiber that lowers cholesterol. However, care must be taken when eating grains in the form of flour. Too many baked flour products—even those made from whole grains—can cause stagnation in the intestines and digestive tract.

The roots of vegetables grow below the ground under the influence of heaven's force. They activate and energize the lower body, including the bladder, intestines, sexual organs, and legs. They are good for strengthening physical and sexual vitality. Roots absorb nutrients from the soil, similar to the way the intestines absorb nutrients from daily food. Conversely, the branched leafy portion of a vegetable grows upward due to the influence of earth's expanding energy. Leafy greens nourish the upper body, including the lungs. Leaves perform a respiratory function for plants, just as the lungs do in our bodies. In order to receive a balanced mix of upward and downward energy, try to obtain carrots, daikon, turnips, and other root vegetables along with their leafy green tops. Both sections can be cooked in the same dish or separately. Contracted greens such as these match the condensed energy of the lungs and large intestine more closely than those with broader, expanded leaves. Among these vegetables, carrots and their tops are especially good for the lungs and large intestine.

Sea vegetables restore strength and flexibility to the small and large intestines, and can be included daily in soups, side dishes, grains, beans, and condiments. One variety, known as agar-agar, is a good natural laxative. Agar-agar is processed into light translucent bars, flakes, or powder, and is used in making a delicious gelatin-like dish known as *kanten*. Agar-agar is first dissolved in hot water and then poured over fruit, vegetables, beans or nuts. Kanten is a delicious natural dessert that is especially refreshing in summer.

Kidneys and Bladder (Floating or Water Energy)

The kidneys have a solid and compact structure that is counterbalanced by the hollow and expanded bladder. The left kidney is charged by heaven's downward force, and the right, by earth's expanding energy. On the whole, the energy that charges these organs "floats" between heaven and earth in the way that water does. The kidneys and bladder are closely related to the functioning of the sexual organs.

Seasonal and Daily Correspondence The kidneys and bladder correspond to winter and night, times when floating energy predominates in the atmosphere.

Mental/Emotional Correspondence Imbalance in the kidneys produces the tendency toward fear. Disturbance in the bladder leads to timidity or cowardice.

Dietary Adjustments Dietary extremes cause a variety of imbalances in these organs. Too many animal fats clog the fine network of capillaries and specialized cells, or nephrons, in the kidneys that filter and cleanse the blood. Moreover, toxic by-products produced by the breakdown of animal proteins build up in the kidneys and damage these delicate cells. Excess sugar turns into fat that accumulates in the kidneys, and so the intake of cake, candy, chocolate, ice cream, and soft drinks can also interfere with the functioning of these cells.

Drinking too much also taxes the kidneys and bladder. People often drink more than they need. For example, a habit such as exercising in the hot sun and then drinking plenty of cold liquid stresses the kidneys and circulatory system. The result can be fatigue, tiredness, or the development of eyebags and other signs of kidney trouble. Theories that recommend drinking a certain amount of fluid each day to "flush" and cleanse the system also contribute to the tendency to overdrink. However, if we eat a naturally balanced diet and drink according to our need, our system will not accumulate toxins nor require "flushing" to remove wastes. The kidneys are also sensitive to cold. The intake of iced or chilled drinks and foods like ice cream accelerates the hardening and calcification of fat in these organs, and can lead to kidney or bladder stones.

The kidneys are also sensitive to salt. When used properly, high-quality, mineral-rich sea salt has a milder, less harsh effect on the kidneys than refined table salt. However, it is best to use salt—even the best natural sea salt—in moderation. The overuse of sea salt, condiments, or seasonings leads to tightness in the kidneys and throughout the body, along with fluid retention that contributes to a puffy or swollen appearance, and to frequent urination, including urinating during the night.

Among whole natural foods, beans correspond to water energy and were used by traditional healers to strengthen the kidneys and bladder. Low-fat varieties such as azuki, chick-peas, lentils, and black soybeans are especially good and can be included daily, as can naturally processed soybean foods such as tofu, dried tofu, and tempeh. A variety of other beans—such as pinto, navy, and kidney—can be eaten on occasion.

A variety of macrobiotic drinks and home health-care practices also help restore health to the kidneys and bladder. Azuki bean tea, which is easy to make at home, helps restore balance in these organs. (Instructions for preparing it are presented later in the chapter.) Azuki bean tea can be enjoyed by those with weak kidneys several times per week for about a month. The leftover beans can also be recycled and added to other dishes.

Hot ginger compresses also energize and activate the kidneys. (See below for instructions on making the ginger compress.) Apply ginger compresses to the middle back several times a week for several weeks in order to strengthen the kidneys. The ginger compress is fine for use by normally healthy adults as a part of home health care. However, it should not be used in cases of fever or inflammation. Persons with cancer or serious illness should use a milder application, such as a hot towel compress, unless otherwise advised by a qualified macrobiotic teacher.

Calluses on the ball of the foot in the area where the kidney meridian begins contribute to stagnation in the kidneys. Soaking the feet in hot water or ginger water can be helpful in softening these deposits and releasing blocked energy in the meridian. It also stimulates the toes, including the fifth toe, which corresponds to the bladder meridian. Soaking the feet in hot ginger water is an excellent way to soften calluses and can be done whenever you do a ginger compress. A nightly foot soak in plain hot water is also recommended for those who would like to soften calluses on the bottoms of the feet. It is also helpful to walk barefoot on the grass, beach, or soil whenever the weather permits. This allows earth's force to charge the meridians on the toes and bottoms of the feet without the interference of shoes, and activates and stimulates their corresponding organs.

Medicinal Uses of Foods

Many people have studied the relationship between food and health, and may already be guiding others in choosing the right kinds of foods to recover from illness and make their lives happier and more orderly. Yet many people still think that sometimes food does not matter so much, or that food is not the answer to certain problems.

That kind of thinking is based on a lack of true understanding of food. If you do not know what kind of food has caused a certain condition, or what kind of food would help alleviate that condition, naturally you may conclude that food is not the issue, and go on to try various other approaches to solve the problem.

Of course, problems always exist on many levels: we can see problems from a medical or psychological level, from a social or emotional level, or from a spiritual level; there are an infinite number of viewpoints as to the cause and correct treatment of human problems, and we can freely incorporate any of those viewpoints. But from a universal, comprehensive, or holistic view, we can always see that all of those things are directly related to food. Food is always the key, central issue, no matter what other types of approaches may seem to help.

It is therefore crucial that we understand the importance of food in our lives, not only on the physical level, but also on the emotional, psychological, spiritual, and social levels. Thousands of years ago, here and there, some people attained universal consciousness and came to that conclusion; based upon their teachings, the way of eating according to the order of the universe was introduced into all disciplines as the base, whether in spiritual life, artistic life, physical or martial arts training, or family life. Food became the foundation for all human activities. But since that time, this foundation has been forgotten, so all of these disciplines, including the art of healing, have become confused and complicated. Now the time has come to recover that simple, basic, universal understanding, and to reintroduce the principles of food into all aspects of human society.

Let us now examine the traditional use of foods within the standard macrobiotic diet for specific healing purposes, beginning with cereal grains.

Cereal Grains

Modern researchers are discovering that whole cereal grains contain many beneficial substances that inhibit disease and promote health. In the field of cancer research, for example, studies show that, as a part of a balanced diet, whole grains, which are rich in fiber and bran, protect against nearly all forms of cancer. In 1981, a researcher at the Louisiana State University Medical Center reported a worldwide association between low death rates from cancer of the colon, breast, and prostate and a high per capita consumption of rice, sweet corn (maize), and beans. Thirty-two worldwide studies have associated consumption of high-fiber grains and grain products with lowered rates of colon cancer. Laboratory studies also show that cereal grains have a cancer-protective effect. For example, rice bran, the outer coating of brown rice, has been shown in animal experiments to reduce the incidence of cancer in the large intestine. Japanese scientists have isolated several substances in rice bran that have cancer-inhibiting properties, and have found that these substances suppressed the growth of solid tumors in mice. Brown rice, barley, wheat, oats, rye, corn, and other whole cereals contain compounds known as *protease inhibitors* that are believed to suppress the action of proteases, enzymes suspected of promoting cancer. Protease inhibitors may also interfere with the activity of oncogenes, which, under certain circumstances, are thought to stimulate normal cells to turn cancerous.

Researchers at the Harvard School of Public Health have experimented with protease inhibitors and have found that they prevent cancer cells damaged by carcinogens from turning cancerous, and cause carcinogen-damaged cells to return to normal. According to Dr. Walter Troll, a professor of environmental medicine at New York University who has done extensive research on protease inhibitors, eating foods rich in these substances can inhibit the development of cancer even in the later stages of the disease.

Brown Rice Traditional healers used brown rice to help eye inflammation, glaucoma, bloodshot, and similar eye disorders. In terms of energy, these symptoms are Jitsu, that is, full of excessive energy, or something like a fire nature condition. If we take usual pressure-cooked rice, that would only make the energy level increase, and not help the problem. Instead, traditional healers soaked the rice in water, drained it until dry, and again added a little water, making something like a soft, uncooked gruel. The gruel was then mashed in a suribachi, with a small amount of added water, and kneaded or pounded into a dough, like uncooked bread or mochi. Even with that pounding energy, there is still no fire or heat used. A small volume of this pounded, raw soaked rice was eaten for four or five days to relieve the eye problems mentioned above.

Sweet Brown Rice This glutinous variety of brown rice was used to heal diarrhea, stomach troubles, and intestinal disorders arising from excessive expanding energy that makes the tissues in these organs soft and watery. To offset this condition, traditional healers recommended using a small volume of azuki beans and a little salt, mixed in with sweet brown rice, cooked soft and pounded into mochi.

Barley In the summer we need a drink that can refresh us;

also in the summer, we should take out any excess animal foods that may have been stored within our body, to better adapt to the heat. For those purposes, traditional healers used barley, which was widely known for its properties in offsetting the effects of animal food. They would lightly roast barley and boil it to make tea. Barley tea can be used as a regular beverage.

To offset or discharge all animal foods, the most effective food is a particular type of barley called *pearl barley*. ("Pearled" barley, which means barley which has had the outermost hull layers lightly rubbed or "pearled" off, is not the barley we are referring to.) Real pearl barley is not common today; true pearl barley is not elongated, like wheat, but round, looking something like a real pearl. Pearl barley is available in natural food stores and some Oriental markets. Pearl barley is an effective medicine for someone who has a tumor caused by eating meat, eggs, or cheese, such as many forms of yang cancer. Moles, warts, and calluses are all caused by excessive animal food consumption; to relieve those symptoms, pearl barley can be eaten as a grain dish, or roasted and boiled as a tea. If you take that tea every day, then one by one, moles, warts, and other skin growths will begin to drop off. In general, all problems caused by animal protein and animal fat can be helped by eating pearl barley.

Corn Corn grits are useful for kidney problems, especially when someone is retaining water because of contracted kidneys. The best way to prepare corn grits for that purpose is to simply boil them in water, making a soft cereal.

Corn silk is strongly yin; for certain yang conditions, such as yang constipation or difficulty in urinating caused by eating too much animal food or salt, you can dry out corn silk and brew it as a tea. Yang constipation, by the way, usually arises relatively quickly and lasts a fairly short time; yin constipation is a more chronic, long-lasting condition; these two types of constipation need to be treated in opposite ways. Corn silk tea can actually be used for any type of over-yang condition, particularly in the intestines, kidneys, and bladder.

Buckwheat Traditional healers classified buckwheat as a water energy food, the opposite of corn, which was classified as fire energy. We identify water energy with cold climates, like that in Russia, and with the winter season. Water energy counters or offsets fire energy. Thus buckwheat is helpful in controlling or reducing high blood pressure resulting from too much sugar, fruit, alcohol, or other forms of strong yin. Buckwheat is also good for contracting the tissues of the large intestines, as in the case of yin constipation, making bowel movements regular.

Raw buckwheat flour is good for eliminating worms and parasites from the body. For that purpose, you can simply grind buckwheat into a flour and mix it slowly with water, eating that as raw buckwheat cream. This dish was also one of the staple foods of the Sen-Nin, people who lived in the mountains and practiced a disciplined, principled way of life to gain extraordinary spiritual and physical powers.

Beans, Seeds, and Nuts

Epidemiological studies indicate that regular consumption of pulses (the edible seeds of certain pod-bearing plants), such as lentils, reduces the risk of cancer. In addition, soybeans, a major source of protein in the macrobiotic diet, have been singled out as especially effective in reducing tumors. As with whole grains, protease inhibitors are the active ingredients in soybeans. Laboratory tests show that adding soybeans and certain other beans and seeds containing these inhibitors to the diet prevents the development of breast, stomach, colon, liver, and skin tumors. Whole soybeans and soybean products, including miso, tamari soy sauce, tofu, tempeh, and natto, are staples of the macrobiotic diet.

In 1981, Japan's National Cancer Center reported that people who eat miso soup daily are 33 percent less likely to develop stomach cancer and have 19 percent less cancer at other sites than those who never eat miso soup. The 13-year study, involving about 265,000 men and women over forty, also found that those who never ate miso soup had a 43 percent higher death rate from coronary heart disease than those who consumed miso soup daily. Those who abstained from miso also had 29 percent more fatal strokes, 3.5 times more deaths resulting from high blood pressure, and higher mortality from all other causes.

Black soybeans Black soybeans are good for asthma and coughing, and also for the reproductive organs, both male and female. The proper way of cooking black beans is a little tricky, and requires some patience.

Black soybeans are washed and soaked in a slightly different way than other beans because of their soft skins. To wash, first dampen a clean kitchen towel. Place the beans in the towel and cover completely. Roll the bean-filled towel back and forth several times to rub off dust and soil. Place the beans in a bowl, dampen the towel again, and repeat. This can be done two or three times until the beans are clean.

After washing the beans, place them in a bowl. Add about three cups of water for each cup of beans, and a quarter teaspoon of sea salt. Soak the beans six to eight hours or overnight. Place the beans in a pot, together with the salt-seasoned soaking water, and bring to a boil. Do not cover. Reduce the flame to medium-low, and simmer until the beans are about 90 percent done, which may take two or three hours. During cooking you may need to add water occasionally, but add only enough to just cover the beans each time.

As the beans cook, a gray foam will rise to the surface. Skim off and discard. Repeat until the foam no longer appears. When the beans are about 90 percent done, add several drops of tamari soy sauce. Do not mix. You may, however, gently shake the pot up and down several times to mix the beans and coat them with juice, which will make the skins shine. Continue cooking until no liquid remains.

Azuki beans Traditional macrobiotic healers valued azuki beans for their properties in strengthening the kidneys. There are other special uses for azuki beans. First, they can help regulate bowel movements, making elimination smooth and regular. Also, when someone was bitten by a dog, rat, or other animal, azuki beans were used to help neutralize the poisonous effects of the animal bite. Traditional healers would grind raw azuki beans into a powder and mix the powder with hot water. They would continue giving that mixture for at least four or five days, to make sure the poisonous effects of the bite were counteracted.

Azuki beans are also useful for regulating menstruation; if someone has irregular menstrual activity, or cramps then she can include a small serving of cooked azuki beans daily.

Sesame seeds Gomashio, or sesame salt, is used often as a condiment in the macrobiotic diet. Gomashio has many medicinal uses of its own. But sesame seeds themselves were used traditionally to make the hair darker. Traditional healers would grind the seeds until they were half crushed, and boil them in water to make a tea. They recommended drinking two or three cups of tea every day; then after several weeks, a person's hair frequently started to become darker. This special tea was also found to be helpful in improving eyesight. Black sesame seeds are ideal for this tea, but tan seeds will also work; you can use about two teaspoonfuls of seeds for each cup of water, and boil for 20 to 25 minutes.

Peanuts Because of their oil content, peanuts are not so advisable for day to day eating. When eaten in excess, they can contribute to elevated blood pressure, nosebleeds, and other yin symptoms. When we do eat peanuts, they should be lightly roasted and salted. However, in some cases, they are helpful when taken as snacks between meals. Peanuts can be helpful in cases of diabetes. A diabetes patient can take a small volume of peanuts, lightly roasted and salted, every day as a snack between meals. Peanuts are also sometimes helpful for cases of depression.

Sea Vegetables

Medical studies and case reports indicate that sea vegetables can be effective in eliminating tumors. In 1974, in the *Japanese Journal of Experimental Medicine*, scientists stated that several varieties of kombu (a common sea vegetable eaten in Asia and in macrobiotic diets) were effective in the treatment of tumors. In three of four samples tested in the laboratory, inhibition rates in mice with implanted cancerous tumors ranged from 89 to 95 percent. The researchers reported, "The tumor underwent complete regression in more than half of the mice of each treated group." Similar experiments, in which mice with leukemia were treated with sea vegetables, showed promising results. A 1986 screening of sea vegetables for antitumor activity found that nine out of the eleven varieties studied inhibited tumors in animals.

In 1984, medical researcher Jane Teas and associates at the Harvard School of Public Health reported that a diet containing 5 percent kombu significantly delayed the onset of breast cancer in experimental animals. Extrapolating these results to human subjects, Teas and her colleagues concluded, "Seaweed may be an important factor in explaining the low rates of certain types of cancers in Japan." Japanese women, whose diet normally includes about 5 percent sea vegetables, have an incidence of breast cancer that is from three to nine times lower than the rate among American women, whose diet does not normally include sea vegetables. Dr. Teas and researchers in Japan believe that a chemical called fucoidan may be the most potent among the various anticancer agents found in sea vegetables.

Studies of wakame, commonly used in miso soup and in other macrobiotic dishes, have also revealed antitumor activity. Scientists at the University of Hawaii discovered that when injected into mice, dried wakame prevented and reversed lung cancer.

Plants from the sea may protect against radioactivity. Medical doctors in Nagasaki who, after the atomic bombing in 1945, helped save their patients on a traditional diet of brown rice, miso soup, and sea vegetables attested to this. In addition, scientists at McGill University in Canada reported in the 1960s and 1970s that common edible sea vegetables contained a substance that selectively combined with radioactive strontium and helped eliminate it naturally from the body. The substance, sodium alginate, was prepared from kombu, kelp, and other brown sea vegetables found in Atlantic and Pacific waters. "The evaluation of biological activity of different marine algae is important because of their practical significance in preventing absorption of radioactive products of atomic fission as well as in the use of possible natural decontaminators," the researchers concluded in the *Canadian Medical Association Journal.*

~ **Kombu** This sea vegetable was traditionally used to make the hair darker; also, taking kombu every day was thought to increase longevity; kombu cooked with tamari soy sauce and eaten on occasion (in small amounts because of a high salt content) was used to increase sexual vitality.

Wakame Wakame was also used to darken hair; also for controlling high blood pressure and generally for heart disorders.

Kanten (agar-agar) Agar-agar docs not have much in the way of nutritional factors, but is helpful for inducing a good bowel movement in cases of yang constipation caused by tightness in the intestines.

Vegetables

A wide range of studies have shown that regular intake of cooked vegetables, especially leafy greens and orange-yellow vegetables, helps protect against cancer. Shiitake mushrooms, which are used in miso and other soups and in a variety of macrobiotic dishes, have also been noted for their cancer-inhibiting properties. In 1970 Japanese scientists at the National Cancer Center Research Institute reported that shiitake mushrooms had a strong antitumor effect. In experiments with mice, polysaccharide preparations from various natural sources, including the shiitake mushroom commonly available in Tokyo markets, markedly inhibited the growth of induced sarcomas, resulting in almost complete regression of tumors with no apparent toxicity.

In studies conducted in 1960 by Dr. Kenneth Cochoran of the University of Michigan, shiitake mushrooms were found to contain a strong antiviral substance that strengthened immune response. Researchers now theorize that the shiitake mushroom stimulates the body's production of interferon, an immune substance that counteracts viruses and cancer.

Cruciferous vegetables, including cabbage, Brussels sprouts, broccoli, cauliflower, and turnips, are recommended for frequent or daily use in the macrobiotic diet. These vegetables are recognized for their cancer-inhibiting properties. In a study conducted in the 1970s by Dr. Saxon Graham at the State University of New York, the diets of 256 men with cancer of the colon were compared to those of 783 men who did not have cancer. The men who ate the most cabbage, Brussels sprouts, broccoli, turnips, cauliflower, and other vegetables were found to have the lowest rates of cancer. The researchers discovered that the more of these vegetables eaten, the greater the protective effect. Among the vegetables studied, cabbage was found to have the most beneficial effect: eating cabbage more than once a week reduced the risk of colon cancer by two-thirds.

Lee Watenberg, M.D., of the University of Minnesota Medical School investigated cruciferous vegetables and, in a 1978 article in *Cancer Research*, reported that they contained chemicals known as *indoles*. Along with other minor constituents, including chlorophyll, carotenoids, dithiolthiones, and glucosinolates, indoles are believed to inhibit cancer formation. Researchers at Johns Hopkins University now consider dithiolthiones to be potent anticancer agents. According to Dr. Wattenberg, eating foods rich in these substances strengthens the body's detoxification system, or ability to discharge toxic excess. Epidemiological studies conducted in the United States, Japan, Israel, Greece, and Norway have shown that people who eat a higher proportion of cruciferous vegetables have lower rates of colon cancer. These vegetables are also associated with lower rates of lung, esophagus, larynx, prostate, bladder, and rectal cancer.

Beta-carotene, and other carotenoid pigments found in orange-yellow and dark leafy vegetables, have also been shown to have anticancer effects. A 1981 Chicago study found that regular consumption of foods containing beta-carotene (a precursor to vitamin A) protected against lung cancer. Over a period of nineteen years, 1,954 men at a Western Electric plant were monitored, and those who regularly ate carrots, broccoli, kale, Chinese cabbage, and other carotene-rich foods had significantly lower lung cancer rates than did the controls. The study, published in *The Lancet,* reported that men with the lowest consumption of beta-carotene foods had a seven times greater risk of lung cancer than men with the highest intakes. In the laboratory, beta-carotene was found to prevent skin cancer from developing in animals exposed to ultraviolet light, and to inhibit both the formation and growth of tumors. Researchers have also identified other carotenoid pigments in these vegetables that are believed to inhibit the development of tumors.

Daikon Radishes, including daikon, are good for digestion, particularly when you have eaten oily or heavy foods. A tablespoonful of grated raw daikon can be eaten along with white-meat fish, mochi, or fried foods such as tempura to aid in digestion. Put one or two drops of tamari soy sauce on the grated daikon for optimal balance. Grated daikon tea, presented in the following section, is helpful in discharging fats that have accumulated in the body.

Carrots Carrots are useful for improving cases of anemia and for tight kidneys. They can also help reduce swelling in various parts of the body.

Burdock This strong yang root vegetable grows wild throughout North America. It helps promote sexual vitality and strengthens digestive activity; burdock is helpful for promoting smooth urination in overly yin conditions. It can be included several times per week in a variety of dishes, including kinpira. In this dish, burdock is cut into thin shavings and sauted with thinly sliced carrots in a small amount of sesame oil or water.

Burdock seeds have a special use: you may have seen burdock stalks at the end of the growing season when they open and spontaneously discharge the seeds. If you take those seeds, roast them and boil them as a tea, that tea is helpful for discharging tumors. After drinking that tea for three or four days, the tumor will often spontaneously open up and discharge, healing very quickly.

Kuzu This white starch powder is made from the root of the kuzu plant. It is good for strengthening digestion. Like burdock, the roots of the kuzu plant grows deep into the soil and are charged with strong heaven's energy. In the southern United

States where the plant is plentiful, it is referred to as kudzu. It can be used in making soups, sauces, gravies, and desserts, and in preparing a special drink known as *ume-sho-kuzu.*

Lotus root The edible root of the lotus flower plant grows underwater in segmented lengths and has been valued for centuries in traditional medicine for its properties in dissolving mucus and restoring health to the lungs and respiratory organs. Lotus root is light brown in color and contains thin, hollow chambers. It is available fresh (in season) and dried in Oriental and natural food markets. Both varieties can be used in preparing vegetable and other dishes. Lotus root is also used to prepare a tea that is especially good for clearing mucus from the lungs and respiratory passages.

Onions Onions are recommended for regular, even daily, use in macrobiotic cooking. They have numerous medicinal properties. They are good for calming the nervous system, for people who are nervous, irritable, or overly sensitive. Cooked onions are also good for strengthening the muscles, especially for those involved in heavy physical labor.

There is also a very peculiar special use for onions; if you have insomnia, cut a raw onion into pieces and put them under your pillow; strangely enough, you will then be able to sleep soundly.

Scallion and chives Chopped raw scallion is used frequently as a garnish in macrobiotic cooking. Because scallions are charged by upward, yin energy, they are good for neutralizing the harmful effects of meat and other animal foods. They also help bring body temperature up and quickly increase circulation. If you are starting to get a cold, starting with symptoms like chills or mild fever, headache or coughing, then you can chop a raw scallion, mix it with an equal volume of miso, and thoroughly mix them together. Add very hot water to this mixture, and stir into a thick broth, like instant miso soup; then drink. Almost immediately, your circulation should become active and you should start to sweat; you might then want to go to bed or cover yourself up. This treatment is effective for mild colds, using the principle of increasing a Jitsu symptom, using strong yin to accelerate and discharge milder yin. Chives were also used in traditional medicine. Served in miso soup, they are good for stopping diarrhea.

Cucumber Cucumber is used in macrobiotic cooking as an occasional vegetable, usually during the summer when it is naturally in season. It is useful for stomach troubles; also cucumber stem, boiled in water as a tea, is helpful for relieving beriberi, reducing swelling in the legs, and in relieving other conditions. If you have pimples caused by eating fatty meats, cheese, or milk, then you can apply cucumber stem juice or cucumber juice itself to those pimples to help clear them up. The juice from summer melons, such as cantaloupe and watermelon, has a similar effect.

Cabbage Cabbage is used regularly in macrobiotic cooking. For medicinal use, you can boil cabbage leaves for two or three minutes; this is good for strengthening sexual vitality.

Dandelion The roots and greens of dandelion are good for strengthening the stomach, intestines, and generally promoting physical and sexual vitality; you can either cook the whole plant, after removing the flower, or dry it and use it as a tea.

Mugwort Mugwort is the plant used to make moxa. It is sometimes added to mochi. Mugwort mochi is good for anemia or for pregnant or lactating mothers. Traditional healers used mugwort to prevent or treat insect bites. If you carry mugwort leaves with you, mosquitoes will tend to leave you alone. If you are bitten by mosquitoes or other insects, you can rub on the juice from mugwort leaves or stems; this will eliminate the sensation of itchiness and reduce swelling.

Seafood

Oyster Oysters accelerate sexual potency; if you would like to figure out why this is so, study the reproductive activity of oysters, as compared with other forms of marine life.

Littleneck clam Small clams cooked in miso soup are good for jaundice and other yang disorders of the liver. Miso soup with small clams helps promote production of milk in lactating mothers. Abalone and koi-koku (carp and burdock miso soup) have traditionally been used for increasing the supply of breast milk.

Eel Eels are a highly charged fish; they are good for increasing sexual vitality; eel has also been used for maintaining physical strength during hot weather.

Conclusion

Whole natural foods contain properties that we can use for certain emergency or semi-emergency conditions. Of course, you cannot apply these special uses of foods continuously; after a short time, their effectiveness will diminish; in general terms, the person should be relying primarily on their daily way of eating in addition to their own natural healing powers.

But if you do not know the special uses of foods, then you may find yourself having to rely on various medications, operations, or other scientific medical practices. In many cases, those practices were arrived at through trial and error, rather than from really understanding their effects on the body. Then, since an understanding of the energetic effects is not there, in many cases, the drugs and other treatments that are used may cause more harm than healing. Every day people are suffering from unnecessary complications because they were treated for one type of problem, and that treatment caused another totally different problem to arise.

If you study the effects of various foods, and apply your understanding of Kyo and Jitsu and the five stages of energy, then eventually you can gain real understanding and confidence, and change virtually any type of sickness or disorder through the use of food.

More than two thousand years ago, Hippocrates said, "Let thy medicine be thy food, and thy food be thy medicine." The traditional food remedies presented in this chapter can be made at home in the kitchen. They can help relieve many minor aliments such as colds, coughing, skin discharges, fever, and digestive upsets. When properly prepared and administered, these traditional home remedies are completely safe and do not weaken natural immunity. They have been used as a part of preventive lifestyles for thousands of years.

However, the special drinks and other forms of home care listed in this chapter should not be substituted for qualified medical advice when it is necessary. Therefore, persons with serious conditions are advised to contact a physician at their earliest opportunity. In addition, all readers are encouraged to contact a local macrobiotic teacher or macrobiotic center for guidance on the appropriate uses of these natural home cares.

Macrobiotic Home Remedies

Every day millions of people take pills and medications for minor symptoms such as headaches, stomach upsets, colds, flu, and insomnia. The root cause of these problems is imbalance in the diet, in combination with changes in weather, climate, and other environmental conditions. Since medications do not change the underlying cause, these symptoms tend to return again and again.

In the macrobiotic view, symptoms such as these can serve a beneficial purpose. Although sometimes unpleasant to experience, they nevertheless help the body to discharge excess and remain free of serious illness. Minor problems can be managed at home by changing one's way of eating (especially by avoiding the foods that are producing the imbalance), preparing a variety of special dishes, and applying simple forms of home care.

The traditional home cares listed below are best prepared fresh, as needed, and used immediately. Teas should be drunk hot. With the exception of regular beverages such as bancha tea, barley tea, and sweet vegetable drink, it is best not to prepare items in this chapter far in advance of use, in large quantities, or to refrigerate, store, or reheat them. The recipes presented below generally yield one to several servings, depending on the recipe and serving size chosen.

Tamari-Bancha Tea Bancha tea with added tamari soy

sauce helps to strengthen the blood if an overly acidic condition exists. It can also be used to relieve fatigue, headaches due to an overly yin or overly acidic condition, and to stimulate blood circulation.

1. Place one teaspoonful of tamari soy sauce in a tea cup and pour in hot bancha tea.

2. Stir and drink hot.

Ume-Sho-Bancha Bancha tea with tamari soy sauce and umeboshi plum can be used to strengthen the blood, regulate digestion and circulation, and to alleviate fatigue, weakness, and various conditions caused by overconsumption of yin foods or beverages.

1. Place a half or a whole umeboshi plum in a tea cup with one-half to one teaspoonful of tamari soy sauce.

2. Pour in hot bancha tea and stir well. Drink hot.

Ume-Sho-Kuzu This traditional home remedy is good for strengthening the intestinal condition, digestion, and restoring energy. It is also good for stomach problems, and can help prevent the onset of colds and flu.

1. Dilute one heaping teaspoon of kuzu with a several teaspoonfuls of water.

2. Add diluted kuzu to one cup of water.

3. Add the meat of an umeboshi plum to the water and kuzu.

4. While bringing to a boil, stir constantly to prevent lumping. Reduce the flame and simmer until it is translucent.

5. Add one-half to one teaspoonful of tamari soy sauce and stir. Simmer for thirty seconds. Drink hot.

Ume-Sho-Kuzu with Ginger This drink can be used in place of plain ume-sho-kuzu. It has a slightly more yin effect.

Prepare in same manner as above, but add one-eighth teaspoon freshly grated ginger at the same time that you add tamari soy sauce.

Mu Tea This traditional macrobiotic beverage is good for digestive problems (e.g., a weak stomach); for respiratory problems (e.g., coughing); for reproductive disorders (e.g., menstrual cramps or irregular menstruation). Mu tea is composed of a combination of sixteen plants and wild herbs. The drink contains a balanced combination of yin and yang ingredients; however on the whole it has a somewhat more yang effect. A less yang Mu tea, containing only nine ingredients, is also available.

Umeboshi Tea This is a very refreshing drink in the summer. It has a mildly alkaline reaction.

1. Boil the meat of an umeboshi plum in a quart of water for thirty minutes.

2. Strain. If the drink tastes too salty, dilute with water.

3. Allow to cool and drink.

Carrot-Daikon Drink This drink helps to dissolve deposits of solidified fat deep within the body.

1. Finely grate one-third cup of raw carrot and the same amount of raw daikon.

2. Add two cups of water, and boil for three to five minutes with a pinch of sea salt or several drops of tamari soy sauce for taste.

3. Drink the juice and eat the gratings, preferably while the drink is still hot.

Azuki Bean Tea This traditional macrobiotic remedy is good for relieving kidney or bladder problems and easing constipation.

1. Place one cup of beans in a pot and add three or four times more water and a three-inch strip of kombu.

2. Bring to a boil.

3. Reduce flame to low, cover and simmer for forty-five minutes to an hour.

4. Strain the juice through a strainer and drink hot.

Shiitake Mushroom Tea Shiitake tea can be used to help reduce fevers in small children and babies, to help discharge animal foods, to help discharge toxins in boils resulting from overconsumption of animal foods, and to help the body relax from an overly salty or contracted condition.

1. Place one cup of water and one shiitake mushroom in a saucepan.

2. Bring to a boil.

3. Reduce the flame and simmer several minutes.

4. Add a drop of tamari soy sauce and drink hot.

Fresh Lotus Root Tea This drink can be used to help relieve mucus in the lungs or respiratory passages, and to ease coughing. It should be thick and creamy.

1. Wash fresh lotus root.
2. Grate one-half cup of lotus root. Place the pulp in cheesecloth and squeeze the juice into a saucepan.
3. Add an equal amount of water.
4. Add a pinch of sea salt, bring to a boil, reduce the flame, and simmer for several minutes.

Sweet Vegetable Drink This drink is good for people suffering from hypoglycemia, tightness in the pancreas, and stomach and spleen problems.

1. Use equal amount of four sweet vegetables (carrot, squash, onion, and cabbage).
2. Add four times more water than vegetables.
3. Bring to a boil and then simmer for fifteen to twenty minutes.
4. Strain and drink several cups a day.

Kombu Tea Tea made from kombu strengthens the blood, helps the body discharge animal fats and proteins, and helps restore normal functioning in the nervous system.

1. Boil a three-inch strip of kombu in a quart of water until only half the water is left (about ten minutes).
2. Drink several cups per day for several days.

Daikon Hip Bath A hip bath made from daikon leaves and sea salt warms the body and helps restore the female reproductive organs to a healthy condition. It also helps relieve skin problems, aids in extracting body odors due to the consumption of animal foods, and draws out excess fat and oil from the body.

Dry fresh daikon leaves in a shady place until they are brown and brittle. If daikon leaves are not available, use turnip leaves or a handful of arame seaweed.

1. Place four or five bunches of dried leaves in a large pot.
2. Add four to five quarts of water and bring to a boil.
3. Reduce to a medium flame and boil the leaves until the water is brown.
4. Add a handful of sea salt and stir to dissolve.

5. Pour the hot liquid into a small tub. Add the water until the bath level is waist-high when sitting in the tub.

6. Keep the temperature as hot as possible and keep the body covered with a large towel.

7. Soak your lower body in the bath for ten to fifteen minutes, preferably just before bedtime, but at least one hour after eating.

Note: Keep the hip area warm after coming out of the bath.

Tofu Plaster The cool tofu plaster helps concussions, fevers, and burns. In many cases it is more effective than ice.

1. Squeeze the liquid from tofu, mash the tofu, and mix with about 10 to 20 percent unbleached white flour and 5 percent grated ginger.

2. Mix the ingredients thoroughly.

3. Apply the plaster directly to the skin, place a towel over it, and tie it in place so it does not move.

4. Change the plaster every couple hours, or when it becomes hot.

Buckwheat Plaster This plaster draws out retained water or other fluids, and helps reduce swelling in the legs, arms, abdomen, and other parts of the body.

1. Mix buckwheat flour with a little sesame oil and hot water to form a stiff, hard dough.

2. Apply directly to the swollen area, three-quarters of an inch thick.

3. Remove after several hours.

4. As the plaster draws out the fluid, the dough will become soft and watery. When this happens, put on a fresh plaster with new, stiff dough.

Taro Plaster The taro plaster draws out stagnant blood, pus, and carbon from tumors, boils, and so on.

1. Remove the skin from the taro potato.

2. Grate the potato.

3. Add 5 percent grated ginger and mix. If the paste causes too much itching, do not add ginger.

4. If the paste is wet, add some unbleached white flour for a firmer consistency.

5. Spread the mixture on a thick piece of cotton, about a half-inch thick, and apply the plaster directly to the area.

6. Change the plaster every four hours.

7. Before applying the taro potato plaster, a five-minute ginger or hot towel compress can be given to warm up the skin.

8. If the plaster is too cold, place a warm salt pack on top.

9. If the plaster causes itching, rub sesame oil on the skin before the plaster is applied.

White Potato Plaster This recipe can be used in place of the taro plaster, if taro potatoes are not available.

1. Grate fresh potato (green potatoes are best).

2. Mix 45 percent potato, 45 percent finely chopped greens (which have been mashed in a suribachi), and about 10 percent grated ginger. Mix thoroughly.

3. If the potato is very watery, place it in a sack made of cheesecloth and squeeze out excess water before combining it with the other ingredients.

4. It may also be necessary to add white flour to the mixture.

Note: Use this plaster in the same way as a taro plaster.

Chlorophyll Plaster A plaster made from fresh leafy greens is useful for helping the body discharge fever and relieving burns.

1. Chop several green leafy vegetable leaves (collards, kale, etc.) very finely.

2. Place in a suribachi and grind.

3. White flour may be added to the green paste to thicken it if necessary.

4. Spread the paste on a towel, a half-inch thick, and apply. Leave it on for two or three hours.

Ginger Compress The ginger compress helps stimulate circulation and dissolve stagnation.

1. Using a fine grater, grate a baseball-sized clump of fresh ginger root.

2. Place the ginger in a small sack made of cheesecloth and tie.

3. Bring one gallon of water to a boil, reduce the flame to low, and squeeze the ginger juice from the sack into the water.

4. Place the sack in the pot and let it simmer for five minutes.

5. Dip a towel into the ginger water, wring tightly, and apply it to the desired area.

6. Change the towel every several minutes and replace it with a fresh, hot towel; continue until the area becomes red.

Note: For people with a serious illness, such as cancer, do not use the ginger compress for more than five minutes.

This ginger solution can also be used for body scrubs to activate general energy and blood circulation.

Salt Pack A warm salt pack can be used to heat parts of the body (stiff muscles, abdominal area for diarrhea or menstrual cramps).

1. Roast dry salt in a stainless steel skillet until it is very hot.

2. Place the hot salt in a thick cotton sack or pillowcase.

3. Do not place hot salt in synthetic material; the material might melt.

4. Wrap the sack in a thick cotton towel and apply to the affected area.

5. Change the salt when it starts to cool off.

6. Save the salt; it may be used again. However, when the salt becomes gray from reuse, it no longer retains heat and may be discarded.

Afterword

Every year thousands of cancer patients visit macrobiotic centers for dietary and way of life guidance, including cooking instruction. The macrobiotic approach does not conflict with modern medicine; rather it is based on the view that cancer can be prevented and reversed by changing its underlying cause. Macrobiotic recoveries are not miracles; they occur as the result of consciously applying natural law. To understand why macrobiotic living can bring about the recovery from disease, we need to understand the relationship between the visible and invisible, or material and spiritual aspects of human life.

At the turn of the century, cancer affected 1 out of 25 people. By 1950, 1 out of 8 developed it, and by 1985, the cancer rate had climbed to 1 out of 3. The rate of cancer has constantly increased, even though scientific cancer research began more than one-hundred years ago. Until now, cancer research has focused on treating symptoms, but has yet to discover what causes cancer or how to prevent it.

Modern medicine is largely symptomatic. When symptoms arise, doctors do whatever they can to eradicate them. If a woman develops breast cancer, for example, cancer specialists try to eliminate the tumor by using such methods as hormone therapy, radiation, and chemotherapy. If the tumor disappears, the treatment is considered successful. But these treatments deal only with symptoms; they do not change the underlying cause.

Health is a product of what we eat, the kind of lifestyle we pursue, and the type of environment we live and work in; in other words, our total way of life. However, since modern medicine concentrates almost exclusively on the elimination of symptoms, it does not address these larger issues. In many cases, the techniques it employs to erase symptoms cause people to become further alienated from the natural order. This dilemma underlies the practice of medicine today.

As we have seen, we are constantly receiving energy from the universe. These vibrations enter the spiral on top of the head, and pass through the body on their way to the center of the earth. These vibrations take the form of temperature, pressure, invisible particles and waves, and the fundamental forces of attraction and repulsion found throughout the universe. We also receive energy from the earth, because the earth rotates and discharges expanding force. Earth's force is constantly coming in through the feet and legs, and toward the center of the body through the genital organs.

We receive the energies of heaven and earth in the form of an expanding and contracting, or pumping motion. Our breathing is a reflection of this rhythm, as is the heartbeat. When we breathe in, heaven's force enters the body. When we breathe out, earth's force is being discharged. Heaven's and earth's forces collide deep within the body and create seven energy centers, or chakras. The chakras are places where energy gathers, condenses, and circulates before being discharged. In the northern hemisphere, energy in the chakras rotates in a counterclockwise direction.

Our body does not grow from the bottom up, like a tree, but from the top down. At birth, our head is big, while the rest of the body is small. As we grow, the body becomes proportionally larger than the head. The major direction of growth is downward. Our origin is in the universe, including the invisible world of vibration, and the network of chakras and meridians constantly feeds this energy to the cells.

Modern medicine is unaware of this invisible energy system. Until now, science has dealt exclusively with the visible, physical world, and has had no awareness of the energy constitution underlying existence. That is one reason why medical researchers have been unable to stem the tide of degenerative diseases.

In Oriental countries, sickness is viewed as a disorder of the body's invisible energy system. The physical body itself is viewed as energy that has a more condensed, visible form. From this perspective, we see that each cell is charged with consciousness. Each thought is transmitted to millions of cells. For example, if a woman believes she is pregnant, her belief can cause the uterus to enlarge, even though she is not actually pregnant. If you constantly think, "I am getting an ulcer," your worrying may cause an ulcer to develop. Our thoughts produce actual physical changes in our cells and tissues.

Energy from the earth takes the form of plants, water, and minerals from the soil; all of which we take in in the form of food. These more condensed forms of energy move downward in the body. During digestion, food is broken down into primordial molecules and energy which are absorbed by the bloodstream. The blood carries earth's energy, in the form of nutrients, to all of the cells. The proteins, fats, carbohydrates, and minerals that we eat in the form of food cause the cells, which are composed initially of images and vibrations, to take physical form. It is because of eating that our invisible, spiritual form becomes visible and touchable.

If we take in excess energy because of eating too much, excess naturally goes to the cells. This excess is unnecessary for the functioning of the cell and must be discharged. Excess energy goes to the meridians, and is discharged through the meridian holes, or points, which are like miniature volcanoes. Excess fat, protein, carbohydrate, and minerals enter the lymph system, and are filtered out by the lymph nodes. Other surplus goes to the kidneys, where it is discharged through urination. Some goes to the lungs, where it is discharged in the form of carbon dioxide. The bloodstream also carries excess to the skin, where it is discharged through the sweat glands.

If our intake is roughly equivalent to our actual needs, normal channels of discharge—urination, breathing, bowel movement, and daily thinking and activity—are sufficient to remove whatever minor excess we take in. However, if our intake is excessive, not only on occasion, but continuously, every day, our body has to discharge this, otherwise, the cells can no longer function as centers of thought and consciousness. In order to discharge excess, fats and proteins are transported through the bloodstream to the kidneys. If the amount of excess is small, the kidneys can discharge it. If the amount is large, it begins accumulating, creating fatty deposits and kidney stones. The accumulation of excess in the lungs leads to deposits of fat and mucus, including various types of cysts. When excess accumulates in the lymph stream, the lymphatic system must overwork in order to discharge it, and the lymph nodes become swollen and inflamed. If this situation becomes chronic, it can lead to a condition such as lymphoma.

The accumulation of saturated fat in the bloodstream causes a layer of hard fat to appear under the skin. Hard fats clog the sweat glands, so that the skin becomes dry. In this condition, the person is no longer able to create skin discharges or skin disease, which help eliminate excess from the body. When skin discharges occur, less excess accumulates inside the body. In that sense, they serve a beneficial purpose. The same is true of allergic reactions. But as fat continues to accumulate under the skin, the ability to discharge through the surface of the body diminishes. If the sweat glands become completely blocked, the person loses the ability to sweat.

Excess also accumulates along the meridians, clogging the meridian holes. Accumulated fat and protein, in the form of calluses, may start to appear on the meridian holes, or points, on the toes and bottoms of the feet. The discharge of fats and proteins through the meridian holes is similar to the discharge of thick molten liquid from a volcano. These accumulations lessen the body's ability to absorb energy from the environment, and its ability to discharge energy from inside.

When the skin becomes blocked, a person feels full or stuck inside. This condition is referred to as "stress." However, if we are discharging normally, we do not feel stress regardless of circumstance or pressure.

Stress is actually an internal condition created by the inability to discharge smoothly. If we continue eating excessively, the body's major discharge pathways eventually become blocked. The person can no longer discharge through the sweat glands and energy holes on the skin. The ability of the lymph system to remove excess becomes lessened, and because of accumulations of fat, the kidneys, lungs, and intestines lose their ability to eliminate waste effectively. Excess protein, calories, and fat travel through the bloodstream to the cells, where this constant influx of excessive, high-energy factors can cause the cells to lose their proper density and start to explode. This uncontrolled proliferation of cells is known as cancer.

The Underlying Cause of AIDS

If, among the volume of excess being consumed, the intake of strong yin is especially predominant, a different type of degenerative process may occur. Instead of the explosion of cells that characterizes cancer, the cells start to decompose, putrefy, and break down into millions of viruses. This process is similar to what happens when meat and other forms of animal flesh decay. When eaten excessively, extremes such as ice cream, sugar, chocolate, tropical fruits and spices, milk, and drugs and medications cause cells to decay and change into viruses, including the herpes, Epstein-Barr, and human immunodeficiency virus (HIV). Viruses can also be transmitted through intercourse, injections, or blood transfusions, but at the same time, we are producing them ourselves. We make ourselves decompose by consuming too many yin extremes.

Of the hundreds of AIDS patients I have met, all consumed large amounts of yin, and that initiated the decomposition of cells and production of viruses. These self-generated viruses can then be transmitted to other persons with similar dietary and lifestyle habits, through intercourse, blood transfusions, and shared needles. In the receiver, these transmitted viruses accelerate the decomposition of cells and production of more viruses. However, the underlying cause of this process is the intake of extreme yin. The virus is the result of this process, not the cause.

To recover from virus diseases, a person needs to change his way of eating to preserve his cells, not let them decay. Persons with virus diseases need a larger volume of minerals in their diets. Their dietary balance should be moderate, with few extreme, high-energy foods. Instead of eating plenty of simple sugar, their diet should be based around foods rich in complex sugars. It should include plenty of organic vegetables that are rich in minerals, along with daily servings of sea vegetables. When properly applied, the macrobiotic way of eating can reverse the process of cell decay. As the person begins forming healthy new blood and cells, the symptoms of AIDS gradually disappear.

Creating Health or Creating Sickness

It is simple to achieve good health; it is far more difficult to make ourselves sick. To become sick, we have to eat ice cream, we have to eat steak, and we have to lead a chaotic life; otherwise, we do not become sick. But it is very simple to be healthy. We need not have a chaotic life, but an ordinary, simple, modest life. Many people hate sickness. They feel sickness is our enemy, that it occurs unexpectedly, that we cannot do anything about it, or that it is due to misfortune or bad luck. In actuality, however, sickness is something that we create.

If we automatically changed ourselves to adapt to changes in our environment, we would never get sick. However, we all have free will, or free consciousness. By exercising that free will, we go against nature, against the movement of the universe, and the result of our actions is sickness. At night we should sleep, but instead we stay awake. During the day, we should keep busy, but instead we sleep. In winter we should not take ice cream, but instead we eat a half-gallon. Our free will makes it possible for us to continuously violate nature.

If we discover the source of this freedom, we discover the secret of life and the key to health and happiness. The forces of heaven and earth constantly flow through the body, charging and vitalizing our life functions. Heaven's force comes down but ends in the uvula. Earth's energy comes up and ends in the tongue. Between them is an open space where the forces of heaven and earth are not connected. It is here that we have a valve. By switching the valve off or on, or by opening or closing it, we decide whether these energies come in or not, or whether we take in a little bit or a lot. We use this valve to adjust our intake in various ways, and that is how we manage our freedom. That open space is the mouth.

Our destiny is determined by the way we use our mouths. Whether we experience fortune or misfortune, health or sickness, war or peace depends entirely on what we do here. Through breathing we cope with the ocean of air that covers the earth. Through eating we cope with the products of the earth itself. The energies of heaven and earth collide in the throat chakra, circulate, and are discharged in the form of waves. This is speech. We use our eating, breathing, and speaking to manage our relationship with the environment and control our destiny. All spiritual practices eventually arrive here; for example, chanting or meditating in silence, activating or deactivating breathing, fasting, or eating in a certain way to bring forth different aspects of our spirituality.

Our thinking is also controlled in the mouth. When you think of the past, what kind of posture do you assume? Do you look downward or upward? You look downward. You bend forward and curve your body inward. Rodin's thinker is thus reflecting on the past. Your whole body is a spiral. In order to think of the past, you need to make your body spiral condensed. When you expand or relax your spiral, you are able to think of the future. When you think of the past, how do you use your mouth? Your mouth tends to be closed, and your tongue attaches to the palate. When you think of the future, your mouth is usually open and loose, and your tongue separates from the palate and relaxes.

In the infinite universe, beyond the world of moving phenomena, there is no past or future. There is only the present. In this phenomenal world, there is no present; only yin and yang, future and past. Try to hold the present. As soon as you try to grasp it, it has already become the past. There is no present in this phenomenal world, but only events that have occurred or events that are yet to come. Where does the present exist? The present does not exist in this relative, phenomenal world. The present is the infinite universe itself, which is without beginning or end and which exists beyond our relative universe. The eternal present differentiates into future and past, or yin and yang. Whether we interpret that infinite present as past or future depends on whether we make ourselves yin or yang. If we close our mouths and attach our tongue to the palate, we interpret these vibrations as the past. If we relax the tongue and open the mouth, we interpret them as future events.

Each of us interprets the universe according to our condition. Because everyone uses their mouth differently, everyone interprets the universe in a different way. If we understand that, then we understand why people are different, and can see that differences between people are not good or bad, but a matter of individual freedom. We can also see that what we put into our mouths every day has a decisive effect on whether we are healthy or sick.

The Medicine of Life

In the future, society will embrace a new type of medicine; a medicine based on a unified view of existence. The scope of future medicine will extend far beyond that of modern scientific medicine, and even beyond that of present-day Oriental medicine. The new medicine will embrace the strong points of the world's great healing systems, while discarding or reforming their less satisfactory aspects.

The new medicine will cover many areas. It will not be limited to the relief of symptoms, but will seek to change the factors that cause illness to arise, including daily food, lifestyle, and thinking. Each of these aspects is important. For example, if someone tries to eat well, yet thinks, "I can't recover; I may die," this depressed state of mind interferes with natural recovery. It is important to maintain a bright, positive outlook. Our thoughts have a direct influence on the quality of each cell. Let us now see how macrobiotic way of life recommendations address the larger issues involved in creating health.

To help the body discharge toxins, we need to open clogged pores and sweat glands, and remove blockage that may be impeding the flow of energy. We therefore advise scrubbing the whole body with hot wet towel morning and night, and whenever possible, removing calluses from the feet and toes. A daily half-hour walk is also recommended, as it helps activate circulation, breathing, and the discharge of excess, and releases stagnation in body and mind. It is a good idea to sing every day, preferably joyful, happy songs that uplift the spirit. Singing makes your breathing become better, and activates energy flow. We recommend singing every day.

In terms of diet, we recommend eating fewer calories, and less protein and fat. The macrobiotic diet can help everyone maintain adequate strength while developing a healthy active condition. It is not enough to limit the intake of nutrients, for example, by eating a diet of raw fruit or vegetables; for maximum health we need an adequate—but not excessive—intake of high-quality carbohydrates, proteins, fats, and minerals. In order to utilize the nutrients in whole grains, beans, vegetables, and sea vegetables, we recommend chewing well. Moreover, in order to quickly neutralize the effects of past intake of meat, eggs, cheese, poultry, milk, sugar, and other extremes, we utilize simple home remedies, including special drinks and teas made from daily foods. These simple macrobiotic remedies can be prepared at home with foods available in the kitchen.

Environmental factors are also important. The ability to discharge depends upon such factors as weather, air pressure, and humidity. In order to help the skin discharge effectively, it is better to wear clothing made of cotton and other vegetable fabrics, rather than synthetic materials, and to use cotton sheets and pillowcases. In order to freshen the air in the home, it is a good idea to put green plants in the bedroom and elsewhere throughout the house. Opening the windows from time to time, even in cold weather, helps keep air circulation smooth.

Watching color television, or spending many hours in front of a computer, causes radiation to be absorbed through the skin, and diminishes the flow of energy in the chakras and meridians. It is better to minimize the use of computers or the amount of time spent in front of the television, especially during the recovery period. Keeping active and busy stimulates metabolism and energy flow. The recovery of health depends on four primary factors: food and drink, thinking, environment, and lifestyle, including daily activity. The new medicine will address each of these areas and treat each person in his or her totality.

Education will play a primary role in the new medicine. The key issue in health and healing is whether or not we can change ourselves. In the beginning, most people do not know why or how their illness developed. Study and self-reflection are therefore necessary to deepen our awareness of natural order, and the role of diet, attitude, and lifestyle in health and sickness. It is also essential to learn proper cooking.

Self-responsibility is another important aspect of the new medicine. After we learn how to cook, eat, and orient daily life in harmony with nature, how accurately we put this knowledge into practice is entirely up to us. No one else can do such things as chew, exercise, or wear cotton clothing for us. If we do not apply this knowledge in our lives, or if we apply it in a casual or careless manner, recovery is difficult. Therefore we need to firmly resolve to change ourselves; to change our way of eating, thinking, and lifestyle. We must change our way of life. No one else can accomplish this for us. Everyone is entirely free; no one can control or limit this freedom. Whether we become healthy and happy, or whether we make ourselves sick and unhappy, is entirely up to us. Symptomatic medicine cannot change the cause of illness. Since we are the producers of health or sickness, we are the only ones who have the power to change our direction.

The new medicine will concentrate a large share of its resources on education. It will guide people toward an understanding of humanity, and emphasize the correct way of life for everyone, including the way to develop a positive image of health and peace. The new medicine will teach everyone how to extend love and friendship to other people, and how to establish world peace.

Simple Technologies

The medicine of the future will address symptoms, but will emphasize simple, natural methods of recovery. The simpler the techniques, the better. The methods we use to care for sickness should be economical and easy to apply at home. Before modern medicine developed into a formal system, many traditional healers and country doctors practiced folk medicine. Folk medicine was also practiced within the family; many grandmothers or elders knew how to deal with problems such as fever or pain, and their methods were quite effective.

A number of years ago, I went to central Africa to address a symposium on macrobiotics and AIDS. Several hundred doctors attended, including M.D.s, nutritionists, and traditional village healers. I learned that when native people became sick, they first went to village healers who were practicing traditional folk medicine that was thousands of years old. Traditional African medicine is based on the use of special foods and home remedies made from herbs and minerals. If folk remedies are not successful, the patient will then go to a modern doctor. If modern treatments cannot help, he may then visit a shaman, who employs such techniques as prayer and chanting.

If we study folk remedies according to yin and yang, we can understand why many of them are effective. For example, what can we do for a nosebleed? Nosebleeds arise when the blood capillaries become overexpanded and rupture. If we make the capillaries contract, the bleeding will stop. What substance in the kitchen can produce this contraction? Salt. To stop a nosebleed, moisten the tip of a piece of tissue paper, dip it in salt, and place it in the nostril. Have the person lie down for several minutes with the tissue paper in the nostril. After a few minutes, the bleeding should stop. This is an example of folk medicine.

As another example, suppose a woman experiences bleeding following menstruation. If we leave her condition as is, she may start to suffer from anemia. She could go to a hospital and receive medication to stop the bleeding. Or she could try traditional folk medicine. Bleeding from the uterus means that downward energy (yang) is excessive. If we are able to apply the completely opposite type of energy, the bleeding may stop. She is a woman. Her opposite is man. Her husband or boyfriend thus has a completely opposite quality of energy. Furthermore, what part of the body has strong upward energy? Hair grows upward toward heaven. The direction of movement is opposite to the downward flow of blood from the lower body. Practitioners of traditional folk medicine would take hair from a man, bake it, and use it to make a tea. Tea made from baked hair is an effective way to stop vaginal bleeding. Like other folk remedies, it is based on an understanding of energy balance.

Like traditional folk medicine, the medicine of the future will be based on the understanding of energy. Traditional healers were able to balance energy and relieve symptoms by adjusting the patient's diet, activity, and daily life. They employed foods and simple folk remedies to supply balanced energy and help the body eliminate excess. Future medicine will extend beyond the relief of symptoms and deal with causes of illness; starting with individual diet, lifestyle, and way of thinking.

Planetary Healing

Ultimately, the new medicine will guide humanity toward spiritual awareness. Someone may believe that modern civilization, with all of its conveniences, is wonderful, and that foods such as steak and hamburger are desirable as symbols of material success. In order to realize health, however, we must change the view of life that leads us to act out of harmony with nature. Our whole way of life must change. We must graduate from egocentric thinking toward universal understanding. We need to realize that we are a part of nature, and that we have to adapt and change with it, rather than exploit it for selfish purposes. Self-reflection such as this can lead everyone toward a humble and modest way of life, a way of life filled with love and gratitude.

The medicine of the future will help us to solve the problems of human existence. It will utilize simple, natural methods to treat the symptoms of disease, and will be based on a clear understanding of the psychological and spiritual causes of illness. It will guide everyone toward a way of life in harmony with nature and the universe. As true biological and spiritual change take place, humanity will become a more elevated species. Modern intellectual humanity—homo sapiens—will evolve toward a new species, homo spiritus. This new species will live in harmony with each other and with their environment on earth, and will see the end of war, crime, violence, and degenerative sickness. They will naturally share a sense of brother- and sisterhood, and establish lasting peace. The new medicine will thus lead humanity away from sickness toward planetary health and peace. It will open the door to a new world.

Appendix: Principles of the Order of the Universe

The Seven Universal Principles of the Order of the Infinite Universe

1. Everything is a differentiation of one Infinity.
2. Everything changes.
3. All antagonisms are complementary.
4. There is nothing identical.
5. What has a front has a back.
6. The bigger the front, the bigger the back.
7. What has a beginning has an end.

The Twelve Laws of Change of the Infinite Universe

1. One Infinity manifests itself into complementary and antagonistic tendencies, yin and yang, in its endless change.
2. Yin and yang are manifested continuously from the eternal movement of one infinite universe.
3. Yin represents centrifugality. Yang represents centripetality. Yin and yang together produce energy and all phenomena.
4. Yin attracts yang. Yang attracts yin.

5. Yin repels yin. Yang repels yang.
6. Yin and yang combined in varying proportions produce different phenomena. The attraction and repulsion among phenomena is proportional to the difference of the yin and yang forces.
7. All phenomena are ephemeral, constantly changing their constitution of yin and yang forces; yin changes into yang, yang changes into yin.
8. Nothing is solely yin or solely yang. Everything is composed of both tendencies in varying degrees.
9. There is nothing neuter. Either yin or yang is in excess in every occurrence.
10. Large yin attracts small yin. Large yang attracts small yang.
11. Extreme yin produces yang, and extreme yang produces yin.
12. All physical manifestations are yang at the center, and yin at the surface.

Macrobiotic Resources

One Peaceful World

One Peaceful World is an international information network and friendship society of individuals, families, educational centers, organic farmers, teachers and parents, authors and artists, publishers and business people, and others devoted to the realization of one healthy, peaceful world. Activities include educational and spiritual tours, assemblies and forums, international food aid and development, and publishing. Membership is $30/year for individuals and $50 for families and includes a subscription to the *One Peaceful World Newsletter* and a free book from One Peaceful World Press. For further information, contact:

One Peaceful World
Box 10, Becket, MA 01223
(413) 623–2322
Fax (413) 623–8827

Kushi Institute

The Kushi Institute offers ongoing classes and seminars in macrobiotic cooking, health care, diagnosis, shiatsu and body energy development, and philosophy. Programs include the Way to Health Seminar, a seven-day residential program presented several times a month including hands-on training in macrobiotic cooking and home care, lectures on the philosophy and practice of macrobiotics, and meals prepared by a specially trained cooking staff; the Leadership Training Program, which offers four- and five-week intensives for individuals who wish to become trained and certified macrobiotic teachers; and Michio Kushi Seminars, four- to five-day intensives with Michio on spiritual training, managing destiny, and a new medicine for humanity. Similar leadership training programs are offered at Kushi Institute affiliates in Europe, and through Kushi Institute Extensions in selected cities in North America and abroad.

The Kushi Institute also offers a variety of special programs including an annual Macrobiotic Summer Conference. For information, contact:

Kushi Institute
Box 7, Becket MA, 01223
(413) 623–5741
Fax (413) 623–8827

Recommended Reading

Books by Michio Kushi

Health and Diet

1. *The Cancer-Prevention Diet* (with Alex Jack, St. Martin's Press, 1983; revised and updated edition, 1993).
2. *Diet for a Strong Heart* (with Alex Jack, St. Martin's Press, 1985).
3. *Natural Healing through Macrobiotics* (edited by Edward Esko and Marc Van Cauwenberghe, M.D., Japan Publications, 1979).
4. *Macrobiotic Home Remedies* (edited by Marc Van Cauwenberghe, M.D., Japan Publications, 1985).
6. *Cancer and Heart Disease: The Macrobiotic Approach* (with various contributors; edited by Edward Esko, Japan Publications, 1986).
7. *Crime and Diet: The Macrobiotic Approach* (with various contributors; edited by Edward Esko, Japan Publications, 1987).
8. *AIDS, Macrobiotics, and Natural Immunity* (co-authored with Martha Cottrell, M.D., Japan Publications, 1990).
9. *Macrobiotic Health Education Series—Diabetes and Hypogylcemia; Allergies; Obesity, Weight Loss and Eating Disorder; Infertility and Reproductive Disorders; Arthritis*, 1985–88).
10. *How to See Your Health: The Book of Oriental Diagnosis* (Japan Publications, 1980)
11. *Your Face Never Lies* (Avery Publishing Group, 1983).

12. *The Macrobiotic Approach to Cancer* (with Edward Esko, Avery Publishing Group, revised edition, 1991).

Philosophy and Way of Life

1. *One Peaceful World* (with Alex Jack, St. Martin's Press, 1986).

2. *The Book of Macrobiotics: The Universal Way of Health, Happiness and Peace* (with Alex Jack, Japan Publications, revised edition, 1986).

3. *The Macrobiotic Way* (with Stephen Blauer, Avery Publishing Group, 1985).

4. *The Book of Do-In: Exercise for Physical and Spiritual Development* (Japan Publications, 1979).

5. *Macrobiotic Palm Healing: Energy at Your Finger-Tips* (with Olivia Oredson Saunders, Japan Publications, 1988).

6. *On the Greater View* (Avery Publishing Group, 1986).

7. *Food Governs Your Destiny: The Teachings of Namboku Mizuno* (with Aveline Kushi and Alex Jack, Japan Publications, 1986).

8. *The Gentle Art of Making Love* (with Edward and Wendy Esko, Avery Publishing Group, 1990).

9. *Other Dimensions: Exploring the Unexplained* (with Edward Esko, Avery Publishing Group, 1991).

10. *Nine Star Ki* (with Edward Esko, One Peaceful World Press, 1991).

11. *The Gospel of Peace: Jesus's Teachings of Eternal Truth* (with Alex Jack, Japan Publications, 1992).

12. *Forgotten Worlds* (with Edward Esko, One Peaceful World Press, 1992).

13. *The Teachings of Michio Kushi* (with Edward Esko, One Peaceful World Press, 1993).

Books by Aveline Kushi

Cooking

1. *Aveline Kushi's Complete Guide to Macrobiotic Cooking for Health, Harmony, and Peace* (with Alex Jack, Warner Books, 1985).

2. *Aveline Kushi's Introducing Macrobiotic Cooking* (with Wendy Esko, Japan Publications, 1987).

3. *The Changing Seasons Macrobiotic Cookbook* (with Wendy Esko, Avery Publishing Group, 1985).

4. *How to Cook with Miso* (Japan Publications, 1979).

5. *Macrobiotic Family Favorites* (with Wendy Esko, Japan Publications, 1987).

6. *The Macrobiotic Cancer Prevention Cookbook* (with Wendy Esko, Avery Publishing Group, 1988).

7. *Macrobiotic Food and Cooking Series—Diabetes and Hypoglycemia; Allergies; Obesity, Weight Loss and Eating Disorder; Infertility and Reproductive Disorders; Arthritis; Stress and Hypertension* (with various editors, Japan Publications, 1985–88).

8. *Aveline Kushi's Wonderful World of Salads* (with Wendy Esko, Japan Publications, 1989).

9. *The Quick and Natural Macrobiotic Cookbook* (with Wendy Esko, Contemporary Books, 1989).

10. *The Good Morning Macrobiotic Breakfast Book* (with Wendy Esko, Avery Publishing Group, 1991).

11. *The New Pasta Cuisine: Low-fat Noodle and Pasta Dishes from around the World* (with Wendy Esko, Japan Publications, 1991).

Family Health

1. *Macrobiotic Pregnancy and Care of the Newborn* (with Michio Kushi; edited by Edward and Wendy Esko, Japan Publications, 1984).

2. *Macrobiotic Child Care and Family Health* (with Michio Kushi; edited by Edward and Wendy Esko, Japan Publications, 1986).

3. *Lessons of Night and Day* (Avery Publishing Group, 1985).

Philosophy and Way of Life

1. *Aveline: The Life and Dream of the Woman Behind Macrobiotics Today* (with Alex Jack, Japan Publications, 1988).

2. *Diet for Natural Beauty* (with Wendy Esko and Maya Tiwari, Japan Publications, 1991).

3. *Thirty Days* (with Tom Monte, Japan Publications, 1991).

Books by Other Authors

1. Aihara, Herman. *Basic Macrobiotics* (Japan Publications, 1985).

2. Benedict, Dirk. *Confessions of a Kamikaze Cowboy* (Avery Publishing Group, 1991).

3. Brown, Virginia, with Susan Stayman. *Macrobiotic Miracle: How a Vermont Family Overcame Cancer* (Japan Publications, 1985).

4. Dufty, William. *Sugar Blues* (Warner Books, 1975).

5. Esko, Edward. *Healing Planet Earth* (One Peaceful World Press, 1992).

6. Esko, Edward. *Notes from the Boundless Frontier* (One Peaceful World Press, 1992).

7. Esko, Edward and Wendy. *Macrobiotic Cooking for Everyone* (Japan Publications, 1980).

8. Esko, Edward, editor. *Doctors Look at Macrobiotics* (Japan Publications, 1988).

9. Faulkner, Hugh. *Physician Heal Thyself* (One Peaceful World Press, 1992).

10. Heidenry, Carolyn. *An Introduction to Macrobiotics*

(Avery Publishing Group, 1987).

11. Heidenry, Carolyn. *Making the Transition to a Macrobiotic Diet* (Avery Publishing Group, 1987).

12. Ineson, John. *The Way of Life: Macrobiotics and the Spirit of Christianity* (Japan Publications, 1986).

13. Jack, Alex. *Let Food Be Thy Medicine* (One Peaceful World Press, 1991).

14. Jack, Alex. *The New Age Dictionary* (Japan Publications, 1990).

15. Jack, Alex. *Out of Thin Air: A Satire on Owls and Ozone, Beef and Biodiversity, Grains and Global Warming* (One Peaceful World Press, 1993).

16. Jack, Alex and Gale. *Amber Waves of Grain: American Macrobiotic Cooking* (Japan Publications, 1992).

17. Jack, Alex and Gale. *Promenade Home: Macrobiotics and Women's Health* (Japan Publications, 1988).

18. Kohler, Jean and Mary Alice. *Healing Miracles from Macrobiotics* (Parker, 1979).

19. Lalumiere, Guy. *Macobiotic Home Food Processing* (One Peaceful World Press, 1993).

20. Nussbaum, Elaine. *Recovery: From Cancer to Health through Macrobiotics* (Avery Publishing Group, 1992).

21. Ohsawa, Lima. *Macrobiotic Cuisine* (Japan Publications, 1984).

22. Sergel, David. *The Macrobiotic Way of Zen Shiatsu* (Japan Publications, 1988).

23. Sudo, Hanai. *Fire, Water, Wind* (One Peaceful World Press, 1992).

Periodicals

One Peaceful World, Becket, Massachusetts
Macro News, Philadelphia, Pennsylvania
Macrobiotics Today, Oroville, California

About the Authors

Michio Kushi, leader of the international macrobiotic community, was born in Japan in 1926, studied international relations and law at Tokyo University, and came to the United States in 1949. Devoted to the cause of world peace, he and his wife, Aveline, introduced modern macrobiotics to North America. Over the years, he has lectured and given seminars on diet and health, philosophy and spiritual practice, to medical professionals, government officials, and individuals and families around the world, guiding thousands of people to greater health and happiness. Founder and president of the East West Foundation, the Kushi Foundation, and One Peaceful World and author of numerous books, he and his wife, Aveline, maintain a busy international travel schedule and make their home in Brookline and Becket, Massachusetts.

Edward Esko was born in Philadelphia on October 16, 1950. He began macrobiotic studies with Michio Kushi in 1971 and for twenty years has taught macrobiotic philosophy throughout the United States and Canada, as well as in Western and Eastern Europe, South America, and Japan. He has lectured on modern health issues at the United Nations in New York and is on the faculty of the Kushi Institute in Becket, Mass. He is the author of *Healing Planet Earth* and *Notes from the Boundless Frontier* (One Peaceful World Press), and has co-authored or edited several popular books, including *Natural Healing through Macrobiotics, Other Dimensions,* and *Nine Star Ki.* He lives with his wife, Wendy, and their seven children in the Berkshires.

Index

Please remember that this is a library book,
and that it belongs only temporarily to each
person who uses it. Be considerate. Do
not write in this, or any, library book.

DATE DUE